WHAT CAN I DO NOW?

Preparing for a Career in Nursing

Ferguson Publishing Company, Chicago, Illinois

Printed in the United States of America

Y-5

Library of Congress Cataloging-in-Publication Data

Preparing for a career in nursing.
        p.   cm. -- (What can I do now?)
    Includes bibliographical references and index.
    Summary: An introduction to the field of nursing, its career opportunities, ways of preparing for finding a job, and related activities such as volunteering, internship, and summer study programs.
    ISBN 0-89434-252-5
    1. Nursing--Vocational guidance--Juvenile literature
    [1. Nursing--Vocational guidance. 2. Vocational guidance.]
    I. J.G. Ferguson Publishing Company. II. Series.
    RT82.P74   1998
    610.73'06'9--dc21   98-16118
                                        CIP
                                        AC

Ferguson Publishing Company
200 West Madison, Suite 300
Chicago, Illinois 60606
800-306-9941
www.fergpubco.com

About
the Staff

- Holli Cosgrove, *Editorial Director*
- Andrew Morkes, *Editor*
- Veronica Melnyk, *Assistant Editor*
- Mickey Cohen, Kelly Cronin, Jennifer Elcano, Julie McNamee, Veronica Melnyk, Beth Oakes, Elizabeth Taggart, Nancy Weatherwax, *Writers*
- Connie Rockman, MLS; Alan Wieder, *Bibliographers*
- Patricia Murray, Bonnie Needham, *Proofreaders*
- Joe Grossmann, *Interior Design*
- Parameter Design, *Cover Design*

Contents

Introduction

There are over two million nurses working in the United States today. Most work in hospitals, but more and more are working in less mainstream settings—public health centers, corporations, schools, private homes. Just as the focus of their service can be vastly different, the opportunities available to them as health care professionals are equally diverse. If you are considering a career in nursing—which presumably you are since you're reading this book—you must realize that the better informed you are from the start, the better your chances of having a successful, satisfying career.

There is absolutely no reason to wait until you get out of high school to "get serious" about a career. That doesn't mean you have to make a firm, undying commitment right now. Gasp! Indeed, one of the biggest fears most people face at some point (sometimes more than once) is choosing the right career. Frankly, many people don't "choose" at all. They take a job because they need one, and all of a sudden ten years have gone by and they wonder why they're stuck doing something they hate. Don't be one of those people! You have the opportunity right now—while you're still in high school and still relatively unencumbered with major adult responsibilities—to explore, to experience, to try out a work path. Or several paths if you're one of those overachieving types. Wouldn't you really rather find out sooner than later that you're not cut out to be a doctor after all, that you'd actually prefer to be medical laboratory technologist? Or an occupational therapist? Or a health care facility administrator?

There are many ways to explore the health care industry in general and nursing in particular. What we've tried to do in this book is give you an idea of some of your options. The chapter "What Do I Need to Know about Nursing" will give you an overview of the field—a little history, where it's at today, and promises of the future; as well as a breakdown of its structure (how it's organized) and a glimpse of some of its many career options.

The Careers section includes eight chapters, each describing in detail a specific nursing specialty: clinical nurse specialist, licensed practical nurse, nurse anesthetist, nurse assistant, nurse-midwife, nurse practitioner, registered nurse, and surgical nurse. The educational requirements for these specialties range from high school diploma to Ph.D. These chapters rely heavily on first-hand accounts from real people on the job. They'll tell you what skills you need, what personal qualities you have to have, what the ups and downs of the jobs are. You'll also find out about educational requirements—including specific high school and college classes—advancement possibilities, related jobs, salary ranges, and the future outlook.

The real meat of the book is in the section called "What Can I Do Right Now?" This is where you get busy and DO SOMETHING. The chapter "Get Involved" will clue you in on the obvious—volunteering and studying—and the not-so-obvious—summer camps and summer college courses, high school nursing programs, and student health care organizations. In keeping with the secondary theme of this book (the primary theme, for those of you who still don't get it, is "You can do something now"), "Get Involved" also urges you to take charge and start your own programs and activities where none exist—in your school, community, or even nationwide. Why not?

While we think the best way to explore nursing is to jump right in and start doing it, there are plenty of other ways to get into the nursing mind-set. "Surf the Web" offers you a short, annotated list of nursing Web sites where you can explore everything from job listings (start getting an idea of what employers are looking for now) to educational and certification requirements to on-the-job accounts to nurse jokes. (Yes, nurses are funny, too.)

"Read a Book" is an annotated bibliography of books (some new, some old) and periodicals. If you're even remotely considering a career in nursing, reading a few books and checking out a few magazines is the easiest thing you can do. Don't stop with our list. Ask your librarian to point you to more nursing materials. Keep reading!

"Ask for Money" is a sampling of nursing scholarships. You need to be familiar with these because you're going to need money for school. You have to actively pursue scholarships; no one is going to come up to you in the hall one day and present you with a check because you're such a wonderful student. Applying for scholarships is work. It takes effort. And it must be done right and as much as a year in advance of when you need the money.

"Look to the Pros" is the final chapter. It's a list of professional organizations that you can turn to for more information about accredited schools, education requirements, career descriptions, salary information, job listings, scholarships, and much more. Once you become a nursing student, you'll be able to join many of these. Time after time, professionals say that membership and active participation in a professional organization is one of the best ways to network (make valuable contacts) and gain recognition in your field.

High school can be a lot of fun. There are dances and football games; maybe you're in band or play a sport. Great! Maybe you hate school and are just biding your time until you graduate. Too bad. Whoever you are, take a minute and try to imagine your life five years from now. Ten years from now. Where will you be? What will you be doing? Whether you realize it or not, how you choose to spend your time now—studying, playing, watching TV, working at a fast food restaurant, hanging out, whatever—will have an impact on your future. Take a look at how you're spending your time now and ask yourself, "Where is this getting me?" If you can't come up with an answer, it's probably "nowhere." The choice is yours. No one is going to take you by the hand and lead you in the "right" direction. It's up to you. It's your life. You can do something about it right now!

Section 1

WHAT DO I NEED TO KNOW ABOUT

Nursing

?

Let's face it.

Visiting the doctor and going to the hospital aren't on most people's top ten lists of favorite things to do. However, millions of people all over the country do just that every day and enjoy it! They want to be there—most have even worked hard to get there. No, they're not members of some weird group that likes to eat hospital food and wear paper clothing—they're nurses. Nurses that make your doctor's appointment or hospital stay quicker, easier, and less painful. If you think about it, when you go to the doctor, you spend the majority of your time interacting with nurses—whether in the waiting room, at the main desk, or in the treatment room.

GENERAL INFORMATION

The demand for nurses has skyrocketed over the past ten years. More importantly for you, this growth is expected to remain steady through the year 2005. That's great news whether you're a high school student or still in junior high. Nursing has become a highly respected and extremely important career to pursue. Unfortunately, nursing didn't start out that way. The nurses of today—possibly you in the future—have several founding heroines to thank for the nursing industry's current high standards.

In the United States, hospitals developed slowly in colonial times. When someone became sick, relatives and friends usually took care of them. This was true of the upper and middle classes, at least. If you were poor and sick . . . well, that was a different story. Many poor people who became sick were sent to poorhouses because they had no nonworking family or friends to care for them. Medical care in these poorhouses was often little more than threadbare bandages and infrequent medications. Because these poorhouses were run with public money, medical care and supplies were lacking. There was a vast difference in the quality of medical care given to those with money and those without. The care we often take for granted today was out of reach for many poor colonials.

The first hospital in the United States—The Pennsylvania Hospital—opened in 1751, but conditions were very crude. Although called "nurses," the staff were actually just untrained servant women. Obviously, changes were necessary, and the establishment of the American Medical Association in 1847 was a step in the right direction. However, it was not until 1911 that medical reform and nursing standards were addressed and upgraded.

About this time, Florence Nightingale (1820–1910), the founder of modern nursing, was helping thousands of wounded soldiers in the Crimean War. She tended four miles of beds all day long, caring for around ten thousand soldiers during her time there. In the years after the war, Nightingale began to structure nursing into an orderly, trained workforce.

"While our soldiers stand and fight, I can stand and feed and nurse them."—Clara Barton, founder of the Red Cross

In 1860 she established the first school of nursing at St. Thomas Hospital in London. The school trained hospital nurses and nurses to serve the poor in remote and inner-city areas. Nurses were also trained to teach other nurses to spread nursing practices and expertise as quickly as possible. Graduates from the Nightingale Training School traveled to many parts of the world and continued to train others in nursing techniques. The first U.S. school of nursing was established in 1872 at the New England Hospital for Women and Children in Boston. By 1898 there were schools of nursing in New York City and New Haven, Connecticut. Nightingale's work influenced nursing practices in countries throughout the world.

Along with Nightingale's contributions, the early American spirit of giving played a large role in the further growth of the nursing field. Volunteerism, especially by women, formed a foundation for organized nursing in America. At the beginning of the Civil War, Ladies Aid Societies included nurses who traveled to the front lines to treat wounded soldiers. Over two thousand women from both the North and the South served in military hospitals, hospital ships, trains, and wagons. In fact, though better known for her accomplishments with the Underground Railroad, Harriet Tubman (1820?-1913) served as a nurse during the Civil War. Her special homemade water lily brew helped treat hundreds of Union soldiers.

After the Civil War, interest in nursing grew and, along with the teaching of Nightingale, led to the opening of several nursing schools. The most popular method of training nurses was through hands-on work in teaching hospitals, which led to a hospital diploma for the nursing students. Today, this educational pathway is still available to you and others interested in a nursing career.

Lingo to Learn

American Nurses Association (ANA): *This organization represents the nation's two million registered nurses.*

Anesthetic: *Substance used to keep the patient from feeling pain during surgery.*

Defibrillation: *The application of an electric current to the heart of a patient to treat irregular heart rhythms.*

Dressings: *Another name for bandages used to cover wounds.*

Health Maintenance Organization (HMO): *A system of health care with physicians and professional staff providing care within certain limitations to people who pay to be a part of the health care system.*

Patient history: *A record of past illnesses, injuries, and treatments given to a patient; usually taken when the patient is admitted.*

Vital signs: *Information such as blood pressure, respiration, pulse, and temperature that tell how the vital processes of the body are functioning.*

The increased focus on educating nurses also led to the appeal for nursing standards and regulations. You may wonder why nurses were interested in setting standards and creating regulations that they would have to follow and be judged by. There were two main reasons for this. First, nurses wanted to be certain the patients they were serving were given the correct care at all times. Remember, the concern for the welfare of others is now, and was then, at the core of nursing. Secondly, these standards and regulations would help give nursing the professional status it deserved. In other words, nurses hoped that the adoption of regulations and certification requirements would cause others in medical careers to stop looking down on nurses as unskilled and unprofessional. Although nurses would continue doing the same work, with the same level of commitment as before the regulations, it was hoped that standards and regulations would bring the profession of nursing into the forefront of the medical community as a respected occupation.

To answer this demand, nurses established the first national nursing association—The American Society of Superintendents of Training Schools for Nurses. This eventually led to the formation of the American Nurses Association, which remains today in service to the nursing field.

Other state regulations helped support the effort for standardized nursing. In New York, nurses had to be graduates of training schools approved by the leaders of the state university to obtain a license to work in the nursing field. Still, laws were inconsistent within states and between states. Most states required training but did not specify the quality of training required. Nurses with the same number of years of training often had vastly different skill and knowledge levels.

Like the Crimean War and the Civil War, World War II greatly affected the nursing field. More nurses were recruited during this war than at any other time in history. Thousands signed up for the Cadet Nurse Corps. What a perfect time to graduate with a nursing degree! Again, nurses played a vital role in the treatment and care of thousands of soldiers.

Because of the enormous response of these Cadet Nurses, nursing became a popular field of study for women and men. Prior to this time, women made up almost the entire nursing field. (Although women continue to out-number men in this field even today, more and more men are finding satisfying careers in nursing.) With greater numbers pursuing this line of work, more pressure was applied to have a consistent set of guidelines and regulations for the nursing profession.

In 1970, New York revised its Nursing Practice Act and acknowledged nursing as its own separate profession with its own licensing requirements, educational requirements, regulations, and standards. Other states soon followed. Over one hundred nursing organizations sprang up to meet the needs of that growing population of nursing and nursing-related professionals. As needs for specific medical treatments arose, nurses began to specialize in different medical areas, such as cardiology (treatment of the heart) and gerontology (treatment of elderly patients).

//We must be learning all our lives . . . every year we know more of the great secrets of nursing."— Florence Nightingale

Today, nurses make up 27 percent of the entire health care industry. That's staggering considering that the health care industry includes doctors, lab workers, physician assistants, orderlies, attendants, optometrists, podiatrists, chiropractors, dermatologists, dentists, clinical chemists, radiological technicians, respiratory therapists, physical therapists, speech therapists, and many more professionals.

One of the major developments in nursing today is the shift in where nurses work. In the past, most nurses found jobs in hospitals, but in recent years, there has been a shift to community health nursing (or public health nursing). Nurses in public health settings concentrate on preventing disease and sickness through educating the public, promoting healthy living, and working to make health care accessible to those who may otherwise not be able to get it. These are also goals of nurses in hospitals and doctors' offices, but they are more focused on the treatment and care of a patient after the disease or sickness has occurred. Public health nurses try to curb the numbers of sick and diseased people by increasing awareness of the different threats to good health and helping to prevent the spread of illnesses.

Fast Facts

Known as the "Nurses on Horseback," Mary Breckinridge and her team of nurses traveled the dusty roads of the Midwest to provide complete health care twenty-four hours a day to rural areas for the first time in 1928.

You'll find community health nurses in clinics, labor camps, rural areas, schools, outpatient clinics, and other public institutions. Unique settings and people with various ethnic, economic, and social backgrounds await the services of the community health nurse. These opportunities are increasing and pulling many nurses away from traditional hospital roles.

Hospitals are losing their nursing staff to other areas as well. Home health care agencies continue to have unfilled openings for nurses. Home health care allows patients to spend less time in a hospital and more time in their homes recuperating. Many nurses are turning to home health care for the opportunity to become more involved on a long-term, one-on-one basis with a patient and his or her family. Also, these nurses work independently in most cases, so they are free to make their own decisions about general nursing care without answering to other medical staff.

Finally, from the early days of the Florence Nightingale Training School to the present, nursing has been about learning. Advances in technology are one of the things that make the medical industry and nursing in particular, ever-changing and exciting. Medical machinery quickly becomes outdated. Nurses who specialize in certain areas and keep abreast of technological advances and enhancements are in high demand. Whether it be new treatments in patient care or avenues to prevention of disease, nurses must be continually seeking information about new technology and new ways of treating patients.

STRUCTURE OF THE INDUSTRY

Today, most nurses (about 66 percent) still work in hospitals. About 10 percent of all nurses work in community health settings; another 8 percent work in ambulatory care, about 7 percent in nursing homes, and the rest of the nurses are spread out among home health care, clinics, HMOs, research, rehabilitation centers, schools, corporate health departments, and shared practices.

The trend in hospitals today is cost cutting. One of the ways hospitals achieve this is to shorten hospital stays and perform more procedures on an outpatient basis. This policy reduces the number of nurses needed. As a result, many nurses are making their way to long-term care, home health care, school clinics, and community nursing.

Another method hospitals use to cut costs is to merge several hospitals together to become one larger entity with several campuses. Mergers allow different hospitals to share technology, knowledge, programs, and activities.

Despite often drastic cost-cutting methods, from 1980–90 almost five hundred hospitals closed because of financial pressure and the inability to keep up with new technology because of lack of funds. Of the six thousand hospitals in the United States today, one-fifth are teaching hospitals. These teaching hospitals offer accredited medical residency programs and clinical learning sites for nursing students. Large medical centers (called academic health centers) often combine teaching and research facilities.

Hospitals vary in physical size and in the number of patients that can be treated at any one time. Small hospitals may have as few as 25 beds and large hospitals as many as 2,000. The two major kinds of facilities are short-term general hospitals (approximately 160 beds) and long-term hospitals (approximately 900 beds).

There are also government hospitals, with the Veterans Administration Hospital being the largest centrally directed hospital and clinic system. States, cities, and counties have their own hospitals, and there are many hospitals that provide specific care to specific patients, such as women's hospitals, rehabilitation hospitals, and psychiatric hospitals. All hospitals are licensed by the state they reside in and must maintain certain state and federal standards.

The internal organization varies from hospital to hospital, but some general practices are usually found everywhere. Most hospitals have nursing units that are composed of many different nursing areas. The nursing department in most hospitals is the largest individual department, with many levels of general nurses and specialized nurses. Registered nurses (RNs) direct and supervise licensed practical nurses (LPNs) and unlicensed nursing staff members.

The hierarchy of the Nursing Department usually follows this order: chief nurse, nurse manager, staff nurse. The *chief nurse* (or *executive nurse*) is in charge of the nursing unit and makes all work assignments and instructs the nurse manager and staff nurses. The *nurse manager* carries out administrative duties and helps supervise staff nurses. *Staff nurses* complement the doctor's treatment with hands-on care. These are usually the duties and order of positions, but each hospital may be somewhat different.

Primary nursing style is fairly common in most hospitals. The *primary nurse* is completely responsible for all aspects of a patient's care, although other nurses will treat the patient under the primary nurse's instruction. The primary nurse (usually an RN) consults other members of the medical staff on the overall treatment of the patient.

//Nursing is the art and science dedicated to compassionate concern for health, preventing illness, and caring for and rehabilitating the members of our society."—a registered nurse describing nursing today

Matrix style nursing units are fairly new and involve grouping nurses and other medical staff around special projects. The difference between matrix style and traditional nursing styles is that the nurse works directly with a team on a project-by-project basis. Instead of being just one step in the whole method of treatment, the nurse is involved in the entire process from beginning to end.

Functional nursing is a less common nursing style. This style calls for several different nurses to care for the same patient but with different focuses. For example, John Doe may have a nurse who checks his vital signs and takes care of administering medicines, another nurse who is responsible for making sure the medical machinery is working properly, and another who takes care of his comfort needs.

The style of nursing used by a hospital is dependent on several things. The number of nurses compared to the number of patients, the administration's understanding of the nursing needs, the level of training of the nurses,

THE INDUSTRY, CONTINUED

and the management style of head nurses may all be factors contributing to the style of nursing for individual hospitals.

The hospital leadership is usually the administrator, president, or corporate executive officer. This leadership position usually reports to a governing board of trustees.

If you've ever walked through a hospital, you know that it's made up of a lot of different sections, or units. The physical structure of most hospitals includes clinical units, operating rooms, recovery suites, emergency rooms, intensive care units, treatment units, laboratories, radiology departments, pharmacies, social services, doctors' offices and so on. Nurses can usually be found in almost all hospital units where care and treatment are being administered.

Nursing homes offer another structure of work that may differ from facility to facility. Nursing homes usually have more regular tasks, so there may be no middle nursing manager. A chief nurse and a group of staff nurses make up the nursing team.

Home health situations offer a vastly different structure. One-on-one, long-term care means that the nurse is independent of other staff members. He or she will be making decisions and judgments concerning care without constant supervisory instruction. The nurse is usually given complete control over the care of the patient, along with medication instructions from a physician.

Similar to the home health care nurse, community health care nurses are independent also. No supervisor accompanies these nurses to homes that they visit to offer nursing services. They are employed by public health departments and visiting nurse associations.

School nurses and occupational health nurses are unique in that they are supervised by nonmedical management personnel.

CAREERS

The two nursing career titles you may have heard of before you began researching the nursing field—registered nurse and licensed practical nurse—are the heart of the nursing field. Licensed practical nurses make up 88 percent of caregivers in the United States, and registered nurses can be found in areas from anesthetist nurses to emergency room nurses. You can aspire even further than registered nursing and become an advanced practice nurse. These nurses perform many of the duties normally restricted to doctors. Nursing assistants also make up a large part of the nursing personnel in most hospitals; this is a job that you can start right after you graduate from high school.

Nursing assistants help the registered nurses and licensed practical nurses with routine daily care of patients. Depending on where they are employed, nursing assistants may focus mainly on the physical needs of patients, such as helping them in and out of bed, admitting their paperwork, pushing their wheelchairs, and helping them walk. Some facilities also have nursing assistants who take and record blood pressure, pulse, temperature, and other vital signs.

Fast Facts

A recent study found that 25 percent of registered nurses began their careers as licensed practical nurses.

Licensed practical nurses, or *LPNs*, give bedside care to sick, recovering, disabled, and injured patients in hospitals, clinics, nursing homes, and various other institutions. LPNs are required to have technical knowledge allowing them to perform tasks such as giving some medications, preparing and administering injections, and monitoring the patient's condition. They also record the patient's vital signs, assist the patient, and give general care in the form of wound dressing, compresses, and injections. LPNs serve under the instruction and supervision of a registered nurse.

Registered nurses can work in a variety of settings. The workplace often defines the nature of the work for RNs. The following paragraphs list RNs in specific nursing careers.

Hospital nurses follow the medical care instructions provided by the physician to care for the needs of the patients. This includes giving medications and treatments. Nurses also maintain patient records. RNs in this setting also instruct and supervise nursing staff in the bedside care of patients.

Community health nurses, sometimes known as *public health nurses,* work in clinics, schools, and patients' homes to provide preventative health care, immunizations, health education, and nursing treatments prescribed by a physician.

Office nurses assist doctors by preparing patients for examinations, performing laboratory testing, and overseeing administrative duties. These nurses may also work for dental surgeons, dentists, nurse practitioners, and nurse-midwives.

School nurses give physical examinations to students; provide yearly visual, audio, and scoliosis screenings; and educate students, staff, and parents on child wellness issues.

Occupational health nurses work in businesses, government facilities, and factories to provide treatment for minor, on-the-job illnesses and injuries.

CAREERS, CONTINUED

Nurses also give physical examinations and provide educational sessions about workplace safety and health.

Operating room (OR) nurses, sometimes known as *surgical nurses,* do more than just hand instruments to the surgeon (although that is a vital part of the OR nurse's job). There are two kinds of OR nurses—the *circulating nurse* and the *scrub nurse.* The circulating nurse is a non-sterile member of the surgical team, while scrub nurses assess the patient before and after surgery and assist the surgeon during the operation. Scrub nurses must be RNs with supplemental education for operating room skills.

While RNs, LPNs, and nursing assistants make up the greatest percentage of the nursing field, the *advanced practice nurses* have higher training requirements and more responsibility. Nurse anesthetists, nurse-midwives, nurse practitioners, and *clinical nurse specialists* are examples of advanced practice nurses. These advanced practice nurses have enough training and skill to do many of the tasks that are normally reserved for physicians.

Nurse anesthetists are among the highest paid in the nursing field. They administer anesthetics to patients prior to treatment or surgery. Nurse anesthetists have to pass an additional national certification exam in anesthetics.

The *nurse-midwife* or *neonatal nurse,* takes care of newborn babies and their mothers. The nurse-midwife spends much of the workday talking to and instructing new, or soon to be new, fathers and mothers.

Nurse practitioners take on many of the responsibilities of a general physician. Nurse practitioners examine patients, take their histories, and diagnose and treat common medical illnesses and conditions.

Clinical nurse specialists have higher training levels that are focused on a particular area, such as transplant nursing, critical care nursing, and cardiovascular nursing. Duties for these nurses vary depending on the area they specialize in.

EMPLOYMENT OPPORTUNITIES

When looking for a job in nursing, the first places to check into (and the biggest employers of nurses nationwide) are hospitals. Larger hospitals that are equipped to handle hundreds and sometimes thousands of patients are the best bet, although smaller hospitals usually have fewer doctors and need the services of many nurses. Two-thirds of all registered nurses work in hospitals today. Even though hospitals remain the major source of jobs for nurses, they are beginning to cut back in the hiring of nurses because of mergers and pressure to cut costs.

If the hospital scene isn't what you're after, there are plenty of other employers of nurses. Nursing homes and long-term health care facilities are expected to grow rapidly and employ more and more nurses to take care of the aging population. Doctors' offices, community health clinics, home health care, schools, health maintenance organizations, colleges and universities, prisons and correctional facilities, and disaster relief organizations are just a sampling of the wide variety of organizations that employ nurses today.

Fast Facts

Neonatal nurses (newborn baby care) are now able to help save over 80 percent of all infants born up to two months premature.

And, let's not forget the government. The Department of Veterans Affairs runs over 170 hospitals and 200 clinics. The Department of Health and Human Services, Indian Health Service (IHS), and the National Institute of Health (NIH) employ thousands of nurses at all levels of education and specialty areas. Presently, 5,000 nurses work for the IHS in the western United States alone! You'll also find hundreds of nurses working in Bethesda, Maryland, for the NIH.

INDUSTRY OUTLOOK

Better health benefits everyone—especially nurses! More and more people are living longer and requiring nursing care during the latter stages of their lives. The number of nursing homes and extended care facilities is expected to double by the turn of the century, causing *geriatric nurses* (LPNs or RNs who specialize in caring for the elderly) to be in high demand. Home health care for the elderly should see the fastest growth in employment.

The current changes in hospital care and structure are also affecting the nursing industry. While there will continue to be a need for nurses in hospitals, many hospitals are being forced to cut back on their nursing staff to save money and to reallocate resources. What is contributing to these changes in hospitals? HMOs and other health care facilities are growing and providing strong competition. Also, hospitals are releasing patients after much shorter stays than in the past, lessening the need for nursing care. Nurse practitioners, however, should be in high demand as hospitals replace some highly paid physicians with not-as-highly-paid nurse practitioners.

Technological advances in medicine have also made outpatient surgery a common occurrence today. While this means fewer nursing opportunities in hospitals, it greatly increases the demand for nurses in HMOs, outpatient facilities, and ambulatory surgery centers.

Most nurses entering the field today meet the challenges of new technology head-on by acquiring more education and specific training. As medical technology continues to improve, nurses are challenged to upgrade their training and are rapidly moving toward specialized areas. Unprecedented opportunities await nurses who are highly trained in medical technology and advanced medical practices.

Employment for LPNs is expected to increase faster than average at long-term-care facilities and clinics, but is expected to increase only slightly and maybe even decrease in hospitals. Again, the shift toward outpatient care leaves fewer inpatients who require the care of an LPN. Not only are there more outpatients to care for, federal and state legislation has forced nursing homes to hire LPNs to care for patients instead of other health workers with minimal training.

The health care industry overall is expected to grow twice as fast as the economy in the coming decade. According to the Career Information Center, health care (with nursing making up a large part) will account for one out of twelve new jobs in the United States by the year 2000. It gets better: by 2005, one of every six new jobs will fall under the health care industry. Within the health care arena, nursing continues to grow even as more and more nurses enter the field. Where hospitals are slowing down as the main avenue for nurses entering the field, outpatient and long-term-care facilities are taking up the slack.

WHAT DO I NEED TO KNOW ABOUT

Careers

?

nursing

Clinical Nurse Specialist

SUMMARY

DEFINITION
Clinical nurse specialists *are registered nurses (RNs) who have advanced education and expertise in a specific area of nursing.*

ALTERNATIVE JOB TITLES
None

SALARY RANGE
$40,000 to $47,764 to $70,000+

EDUCATIONAL REQUIREMENTS
Master's degree

CERTIFICATION OR LICENSING
Licensing is mandatory for all RNs; additional certification in advanced practice specialties is available.

EMPLOYMENT OUTLOOK
Much faster than the average

HIGH SCHOOL SUBJECTS
Biology
Chemistry
English (writing/literature)
Mathematics
Physics

PERSONAL INTERESTS
Helping people: emotionally
Helping people: physical health/medicine

"See you later," says Matt Brayton, waving to a colleague as he steps into his office. Matt, a clinical nurse specialist at Vanderbilt University Medical Center, begins this workday by checking on patients who have been admitted during the night. Later, he goes on rounds with the doctors and other nurses. One of his responsibilities on rounds is to bring an expert nursing perspective to the attention of physicians.

"Doctors don't think like nurses," Matt explains. Since Vanderbilt is a teaching hospital, Matt often works with medical residents, helping them learn what he terms the "practical, nonmedical stuff."

WHAT DOES A CLINICAL NURSE SPECIALIST DO?

Clinical nurse specialists are advanced practice nurses, which means that they have education and expertise beyond the level required for registered nurses (RNs). The key word in the definition of the clinical nurse specialist role is "expert." Clinical nurse specialists have expert knowledge in a defined area of nursing, such as medical-surgical, gerontological (older adult), and mental health. Within the chosen area of specialization, they function as expert clinicians, consultants, educators, case managers, researchers, and administrators.

WHAT DOES A CNS DO?, CONTINUED

The National League for Nursing Education first drew up a plan to create the clinical nurse specialist role in the 1940s. The first master's degree program opened in 1954 at Rutgers University; the only specialty offered at that time was psychiatric nursing. By 1970, clinical nurse specialty certification had become available in a number of fields in response to the increased specialization in health care, the development of new technologies, and the need to provide alternative, cost-efficient health care in the physician shortage of the 1960s.

The nurse practitioner role was also developed during the 1960s, principally to provide cost-efficient health care in rural and inner-city areas where there were few physicians. Nurse practitioners usually focus on primary health care and prevention of health problems; they are more likely to be community-based than hospital-based. In light of the current direction taken by the U.S. health care industry (shorter hospital stays, more procedures done in outpatient settings, emphasis on efficient management and cost containment), many nursing educators believe that the roles of the nurse practitioner and clinical nurse specialist are gradually merging. (The other two advanced practice nursing categories are nurse-midwife and nurse anesthetist.)

Clinical nurse specialists have different duties depending on where they are employed (hospital, nursing home, community clinic, mental health facility, home health care, industrial setting, or other). But working as part of an interdisciplinary health care team is basic to virtually any clinical nurse specialist position.

The clinical nurse specialist is expected to be able to see the "big picture" in a way that the staff nurse who is focused on delivering direct care cannot. Patients and their families need an expert guide and advocate in order

Lingo to Learn

American Nurses Association (ANA): *The most important professional society for nurses.*

American Nurses Credentialing Center (ANCC): *The ANA's separately incorporated national certification-exam administering organization.*

Change agent: *The term often used to characterize the clinical nurse specialist's role as an identifier, analyst, and solver of health care problems.*

Direct care: *The part of the clinical nurse specialist's work that involves actual interaction with patients and their families.*

Indirect care: *The part of the clinical nurse specialist's work that is aimed at improving nursing care by interaction with other care providers rather than with the patients themselves.*

Nursing service director: *The administrator in charge of a hospital's total nursing services.*

Preventive care: *Health care with the goal of maintaining health and preventing illness (or identifying and treating problems at the earliest possible stage).*

Tertiary health care: *The high-tech specialized diagnosis and treatment available only in large research and teaching hospitals.*

to make the most constructive use of today's immensely complex health care delivery system.

In addition to making sure that the patient receives the most appropriate state-of-the-art nursing care while in the hospital, the clinical nurse specialist also plays the important dual roles of educator and consultant. Educating patients and their families is the most obvious part of the teaching role, but far from the only part. The clinical nurse specialist is also involved in the professional development of the other members of the nursing staff and nursing students by teaching them about new concepts and techniques in nursing.

Clinical nurse specialists may be involved in the planning and development of nursing school courses or continuing education programs either in the hospital or academic setting. They may be called on to provide an expert nursing perspective for students in other disciplines, such as social work or medical ethics. Clinical nurse specialists are frequently called on to provide health care education for the community at large or for specific sectors of the community (such as manufacturers of medical equipment).

WHAT IS IT LIKE TO BE A CLINICAL NURSE SPECIALIST?

Matt Brayton has been a clinical nurse specialist in general internal medicine at Vanderbilt University Medical Center for slightly over two years now. He became an RN three years before, after deciding that the stories his wife told about her work as a nurse were more interesting than the reports he was writing for a local newspaper.

Matt sometimes says that he has a "nonspecialty specialty," since general internal medicine covers such a broad range of medical conditions—infections, heart diseases, lung problems, gastrointestinal problems, and more.

As a clinical nurse specialist case manager, Matt works with the patient, the patient's family, and other members of the health care team to assess the patient's condition and to create an appropriate plan for hospital care.

Most of Matt's day is spent one-on-one with patients. All the Vanderbilt clinical nurse specialists have been given the role of case manager, which means that they are responsible for quality control and efficiency in the handling of each patient's hospital stay. The clinical nurse specialist assesses every person who is admitted: How sick is the patient? How long will the hospital stay last? What kind of financial resources are available? Will the patient need a referral to a social worker, a psychiatrist, or other mental health professional?

Is the patient here because of a chronic illness that is not being managed well? If a problem is caught at an early stage, it can often be handled without hospitalization. An important part of Matt's job is to educate patients in the management of their illness. Asthma attacks can be avoided, for example, if the patient is taught to use a peak-flow monitor every day to measure lung capacity. Simply relying on "how you feel" is inadequate, as Matt explains, since people can lose 25 percent of lung capacity without experiencing any symptoms. Then an asthma attack catches them unprepared and may result in an admission to the hospital.

Likewise, Matt teaches diabetics to use a glucometer daily to check their blood sugar. People with high blood pressure are shown how to use a blood pressure cuff at home to monitor their condition; those with congestive heart failure are taught the importance of weighing themselves daily to find out if they are retaining fluid, which would be an indication that the heart condition is worsening.

❚❚To be a caring person day in and day out is harder than it sounds."

Anne Luther has similar responsibilities as the clinical nurse specialist for otolaryngology (ear, nose, and throat), a position she has held since 1988. (Before that, she was a clinical nurse specialist in general surgery.) Anne usually begins her day by talking with the intern who did early rounds. Sometimes she finds that her first task of the day is "putting out fires"—a medical crisis, a postoperative patient whose condition has suddenly deteriorated, an unhappy family member.

Because Vanderbilt is a tertiary care facility (a hospital that treats illnesses requiring specialized procedures such as coronary artery bypass surgery), many of Anne's patients have come from Kentucky or Alabama to undergo surgery not available in their hometowns. Anne meets with the patients and their families before surgery to prepare them for what they will experience. She continues to meet with them during their hospital stay and makes post-discharge arrangements; as case manager, an important part of her role is acting as the liaison among the health care team members.

Extensive "preop" education is essential: Otolaryngological surgery often means that the patient will wake up with a tracheostomy—an opening through the neck into the trachea into which a tube has been inserted. A patient with a tracheostomy is unable to speak or swallow.

If the patient will be leaving the hospital with the tracheostomy in place, the patient and family need to be taught self-care (the management of artificial airways, for example). Arrangements need to be made for ongoing home health care and physical therapy. Anne arranges for speech-language pathologists to come to the hospital to begin teaching alternative methods of swallowing and speaking, but therapy generally needs to continue after discharge. Removal of a cancerous larynx (voice box) does not mean that the person will never be able to talk again; it means that he or she will need to learn compensatory techniques for producing speech sounds. Anne is the nurse adviser for the New Voice Club, a monthly support group for people developing "new voices."

FYI

The National League for Nursing Education first drew up a plan to create the clinical nurse specialist role in the 1940s. By 1970, clinical nurse specialist certification had become available in a number of fields, largely because of the increased specialization in health care.

Surgical patients have the advantage of learning in advance what to expect. Accident victims are less fortunate. Another important part of Anne's job is working with patients who have suffered injuries that unexpectedly require them to have their jaws wired shut—a highly traumatic experience, especially when accompanied by other injuries that make it difficult or impossible to speak or breathe normally. Anne delivers oral care and teaches the patient and family how to do the self-care they will need to perform after the patient is discharged.

When Anne first started graduate school (after serving as a staff nurse in surgery and rehabilitation and as a clinical instructor of nursing students), her intention was to go into teaching after finishing her degree. When she realized how much she enjoyed working with patients and their families, however, she decided to apply her expertise in the hospital setting instead—a decision that she has not regretted.

HAVE I GOT WHAT IT TAKES TO BE A CNS?

Anyone going into nursing needs to have a caring attitude and a strong commitment to helping people. Emotional maturity, a well-balanced personality, and excellent communication skills are vital. "You need to be able to forget your personal stuff while you focus on the patient's problem," said one clinical

HAVE I GOT WHAT IT TAKES?, CONTINUED

nurse specialist, adding frankly, "To be a caring person day in and day out is harder than it sounds."

A nurse needs to have the ability to remain calm in an emergency and to accept frequent interruptions in the daily work routine. "You have to be able to juggle and reprioritize and have a high tolerance for delayed gratification," Anne Luther explains.

In addition to possessing the qualities shared by all good nurses, clinical nurse specialists need to develop the leadership skills and expert competence necessary for advanced practice nursing. Because the clinical nurse specialist role is still not understood by some doctors and nurses, he or she must have the professional self-confidence to educate colleagues as well as patients and families. Physicians may be reluctant to recognize the qualifications of the clinical nurse specialist, and staff nurses may be resistant to what they perceive as criticism or interference with their work. A clinical nurse specialist also needs to have the academic interest and ability to do graduate study. A master's degree is required, and a doctorate is becoming increasingly necessary for top-level positions involving research, teaching, and policy making.

In today's health care environment, clinical nurse specialists often find themselves spending a large amount of time trying to sort out problems with cost-conscious insurance companies. Many people, especially those with low incomes, often have trouble getting the health care that they need, and trying to work with such situations can be difficult for nurses, who recognize the need for cost-effective care but do not want to see the quality of care suffer.

An important part of nursing, especially in advanced practice roles, is helping patients to help themselves keep healthy. Empowering people this way is often one of the most satisfying aspects of a nurse's job. Yet when people persistently refuse to make the effort to take care of themselves, it can be very frustrating for the nurse who spent hours educating them only to see them back in the hospital with a medical crisis that could easily have been avoided.

To be a successful clinical nurse specialist, you should:

Be able to handle stress and remain calm in emergencies

Be strongly committed to helping people

Enjoy solving problems

Be able to handle a heavy workload

Have strong communication skills

Be well organized

HOW DO I BECOME A CLINICAL NURSE SPECIALIST?

EDUCATION

High School
If you're a high school student and interested in a nursing career, take a good college-preparatory curriculum that includes biology, chemistry, physics, and mathematics. If a course on human anatomy and physiology is offered as a follow-up to basic biology, be sure to take it. English and speech classes that emphasize communication skills (both written and oral) are also important.

There are often opportunities to do volunteer work at a local hospital, nursing home, or clinic. You might also take a Red Cross first-aid course or join a chapter of the Future Nurses Club to learn more about the nursing profession.

Postsecondary Training
Before becoming a clinical nurse specialist, you must become a registered nurse (RN). There are three ways to become an RN—a two-year associate's degree (ADN) program at a junior or community college, a two- or three-year diploma program at a hospital, or a bachelor's degree (BSN) program at a college or university. All the programs include supervised "hands-on" training in a hospital setting. Since a clinical nurse specialist needs a master's degree (MSN), the BSN is the most appropriate educational route to choose. People who are already practicing nursing with an ADN or diploma and decide to upgrade their qualifications generally need to do additional course work to receive a bachelor's degree before they can enter an MSN program.

Courses in a nursing degree program include human anatomy and physiology, microbiology, chemistry, nutrition, and psychology, as well as nursing theory and practice. If you're in a bachelor's degree program you will also take classes in English, humanities, and social sciences.

Graduate programs for those planning to become clinical nurse specialists offer more advanced work in nursing theory, research, and clinical practice, giving students the opportunity to develop an area of in-depth nursing expertise. Usually, nurses have been RNs in staff positions for several years before deciding to enter graduate programs, but that is not always the case. It sometimes happens that individuals in other professions decide to become nurses.

There are various routes of professional transition. Matt Brayton, for example, earned an undergraduate degree in journalism and worked in that field for several years before deciding to become a nurse. He entered a "bridge"

HOW DO I BECOME A . . . ?, CONTINUED

program at a university nursing school that allowed him to move into an MSN program without earning a BSN first.

After completing his MSN, passing his licensing exam to become an RN, and working for several years as a staff nurse, he was eligible to take certification exams to become a clinical nurse specialist. Since he already had his MSN, further graduate study was not necessary.

CERTIFICATION OR LICENSING

To become a clinical nurse specialist, you must first be a licensed RN. The RN is earned by passing a national examination after graduating from an approved nursing program. All states require RN licensing before a nurse is allowed to practice.

National certification exams are offered by the American Nurses Credentialing Center (ANCC) in various clinical specialties, although not all states require these examinations or recognize clinical nurse specialist status.

The ANCC offers clinical nurse specialty examinations in areas including adult psychiatric and mental health nursing, child and adolescent psychiatric and mental health nursing, medical-surgical nursing, community health, home health, and gerontological nursing.

ANCC certification is valid for five years; recertification can be obtained by exam or continuing education.

WHO WILL HIRE ME?

Clinical nurse specialists work in a wide range of health care settings, depending on their particular area of specialization and interest. They are employed in hospitals, clinics, community health centers, mental health facilities, nursing homes, home health care agencies, veterans affairs facilities, industrial organizations, nursing schools and other educational institutions, physicians' offices, and the military. A few are in private or independent practice.

Information about job openings for clinical nurse specialists is available from many sources. Your nursing school placement office is the best place to start; other avenues include nursing registries, nurse employment agencies, and state employment offices. Positions are often listed in professional journals and newspapers. Information about government jobs is available from the Office of Personnel Management for your region. Contacts you have made through clinical work or involvement in professional societies can be helpful sources of information. The organization that formerly employed you as a staff nurse may be eager to rehire you as a clinical nurse specialist now that you have received your MSN and been certified in an advanced practice specialty.

WHERE CAN I GO FROM HERE?

As clinical nurse specialists gain experience, they become qualified for positions that involve greater responsibility and give them opportunities to have a greater impact on nursing practice. Some people choose to broaden their base of expertise by adding nurse practitioner qualifications to their credentials.

Many clinical nurse specialists become involved in nursing education, research, publishing, and consulting. Some may want to make their voices heard in the current debate on the future of health care.

Moving into faculty or administrative positions is the form of advancement chosen by some clinical nurse specialists, while others prefer to remain in positions that are more direct-care oriented.

A Ph.D. in nursing is becoming increasingly necessary for advancement into high-level research, teaching, administrative, or policy-making positions.

WHAT ARE SOME RELATED JOBS?

The U.S. Department of Labor classifies clinical nurse specialists and other registered nurses with people in the "Health Assessment and Treating Occupations," a subcategory of the much broader "Professional Speciality Occupations" field. Also under the "Health Assessment and Treating Occupations" heading are dietitians and nutritionists, pharmacists, occupational therapists, recreational therapists, respiratory therapists, physicians' assistants, audiologists, and speech-language pathologists.

Related Jobs

Audiologists

Dietitians

Nutritionists

Occupational therapists

Paramedics

Pharmacists

Physical therapists

Physicians' assistants

Recreational therapists

Respiratory therapists

Speech-language pathologists

WHAT ARE THE SALARY RANGES?

Salaries for clinical nurse specialists range from $40,000 to $70,000 and occasionally higher. According to a recent University of Texas Medical Branch survey of hospitals and medical surveys, the median salary for clinical nurse spe-

WHAT ARE THE SALARY RANGES?, CONTINUED

cialists is $47,674. Salaries on the West Coast tend to be higher than in other parts of the country.

Clinical nurse specialists are usually eligible for a good benefits package, including paid sick and holiday time, paid vacation, personal time, medical coverage, 401 K plans, and other perks depending on the employer.

WHAT IS THE JOB OUTLOOK?

The job outlook for advanced practice nurses is excellent, since they are winning increasing recognition for their ability to provide high-quality cost-effective health care. As discussed earlier in this chapter, the roles of the clinical nurse specialist and the nurse practitioner may be merging in the near future as many clinical nurse specialists move beyond the traditional hospital setting into outpatient settings with an emphasis on preventive health care. (Outpatient health centers and a focus on prevention are important cost-cutting measures.)

The fact that the role of the clinical nurse specialist is evolving means that people entering the field should be flexible in their expectations and open to further education to broaden their areas of competency.

Areas of practice that are likely to grow especially fast are those involving home health care (in keeping with the trend of getting the patient out of the hospital as quickly as possible) and care for the elderly (since the percentage of the U.S. population in the over-65 age group is steadily increasing). Rehabilitation and outpatient surgery are also growing fields.

Licensed Practical Nurse

SUMMARY

DEFINITION
Licensed practical nurses *administer direct patient care under the supervision of physicians or registered nurses in hospitals, clinics, private homes, schools, and other similar settings.*

ALTERNATIVE JOB TITLES
Home health nurse
Vocational nurse

SALARY RANGE
$19,122 to $23,900 to $28,234

EDUCATIONAL REQUIREMENTS
High school diploma (generally); completion of state-approved practical nursing program (twelve months)

CERTIFICATION OR LICENSING
Mandatory

EMPLOYMENT OUTLOOK
Faster than the average

HIGH SCHOOL SUBJECTS
Biology
Chemistry
English (writing/literature)
Mathematics
Physics
Science
Speech

PERSONAL INTERESTS
Helping people: emotionally
Helping people: physical health/medicine

"Good afternoon, Mrs. Hayes," a cheerful voice calls out to the sleeping woman in Room 29. Harriette Williams, charge nurse on the Smith Unit at The Washington House, is checking on one of her most critical patients, an elderly stroke victim. Mrs. Hayes, paralyzed on one side and semicomatose, does not respond, but Harriette keeps up a pleasant monologue, bending down close and taking up her limp hand. "I'm just checking to see how you're doing, Mrs. Hayes."

Harriette, a licensed practical nurse (LPN) stares hard at her patient—who has a nasal gastric (NG) tube inserted in her nose and down her throat to provide an airway and a feeding passage—looking for any sign of a response. When she gets none, Harriette gently returns the frail woman's hand to her side, opens the curtains to brighten the small room, checks the NG tube to make sure it is functioning properly, turns up the classical music playing on the small radio next to the bed, and promises to return. "I'll be back to check on you later, Mrs. Hayes," she says, leaving the room and continuing down the hall of the Skilled Nursing Facility occupying the first floor of this high-rise retirement community.

WHAT DOES A LICENSED PRACTICAL NURSE DO?

Licensed practical nurses provide quality, cost-effective nursing care wherever patient care is needed. They work in hospitals, nursing homes and long-term care facilities, rehabilitation facilities, doctors' offices, health maintenance organizations (HMOs), clinics, schools, private homes, and in all military branches. Their duties vary according to each state's Nurse Practice Act and the place of employment, but generally involve basic patient care. Licensed practical nurses provide for the emotional and physical comfort of their patients. They observe, record, and report to the appropriate people any changes in the patient's status. Licensed practical nurses also perform more specialized nursing functions, such as administering medications and therapeutic treatments, as well as assisting with rehabilitation. The licensed practical nurse might also participate in the planning, implementation, and evaluation of nursing care.

In the hospital setting, licensed practical nurses usually work under the supervision of registered nurses (RNs), performing many basic nursing duties of bedside care, particularly those that are routine or performed regularly. They take vital signs such as temperature, pulse, and blood pressure; prepare and administer prescribed medicines to patients (in most states); help prepare patients for examinations and operations; collect samples from patients for testing; and perform routine laboratory procedures, such as urinalysis. They also observe patients and report any adverse reactions to medications or treatments. One of a licensed practical nurse's main functions is to ensure that patients are comfortable and that their personal hygiene needs are met. They give alcohol rubs or massages, if necessary, and help patients bathe or brush their teeth. They respond to patient calls and answer their questions.

The licensed practical nurse may work in any unit of the hospital, including intensive care, recovery, pediatrics, medical-surgical, and maternity, with varying duties according to the demands of the depart-

Lingo to Learn

Anatomy: *The science of the structure of the body and its organs.*

Catheter: *A rubber, plastic, or glass tube used to insert into the bladder in order to withdraw urine; or a tube for passage into a structure for the purpose of injecting or withdrawing a fluid into or out of the body.*

Clinical rotation: *Time spent working on a floor or unit of a health care facility, usually as part of required training for medical health care professionals.*

Geriatrics: *A branch of medicine that deals with the problems and diseases of old age and aging people.*

Inpatient: *A hospital patient who receives lodging and food as well as treatment.*

IV: *Abbreviation for intravenous—going into a vein.*

Long-term care: *Care administered over a long period of time, usually for chronically ill or incapacitated patients, such as those in nursing homes.*

Nasal gastric tube: *Flexible tubing placed up the patient's nose and down the throat to provide an airway and feeding passage for patients who are unconscious.*

ment. For instance, in the obstetrics department, a licensed practical nurse helps in the delivery room and may feed and bathe newborns, as well as give basic care to recovering new mothers. Some licensed practical nurses direct nursing aides and orderlies and may also have clerical duties.

In nursing or retirement homes, licensed practical nurses often serve as charge nurses, taking over many of the responsibilities that registered nurses would have in a hospital setting. Because much of the care provided in nursing homes is of the routine variety, licensed practical nurses are used extensively and are often in charge of an entire floor, with responsibility for the hands-on care of many patients. In addition to providing routine bedside care, licensed practical nurses in nursing homes—fast becoming the largest employer of licensed practical nurses after hospitals—may also help to evaluate residents' needs, develop care treatment plans, and supervise nursing aides. In addition, they are charged with contacting doctors when necessary, completing any associated paperwork, and reporting to doctors or registered nurses on patients' status. Doctors and registered nurses often depend on detailed reporting from licensed practical nurses to accurately maintain patient records and treatment course. Licensed practical nurses frequently act as supervisors of nursing assistants in nursing homes.

Licensed practical nurses working in clinics for physicians and dentists, including HMOs, help prepare patients for examination and even help the physician conduct the exam. They apply dressings, explain prescribed treatments or health measures, schedule appointments, keep records, and perform other clerical duties. Licensed practical nurses who work in home health care as private duty nurses prepare meals for their patients, keep rooms orderly, and teach family members simple nursing tasks as part of patient care.

WHAT IS IT LIKE TO BE A LICENSED PRACTICAL NURSE?

Harriette Williams, LPN, has been working in geriatric health care for twenty years, most of that time in the Skilled Nursing Facility at The Washington House, a continuing care retirement community sponsored by the Arlington Hospital Association in northern Virginia. It is hard to imagine that she would ever leave, given the bonds she has forged there, both with her patients and co-workers. "We are a tight-knit family here," she explains, "and often the last stop for patients sent to us. It is our job to take care of them and make them as comfortable as possible until their time comes. You get real close."

WHAT IS IT LIKE TO BE A . . . ?, CONTINUED

Harriette is in charge of the twenty-eight-bed Smith Unit, one of three units providing professional nursing care for resident patients. Her unit receives the neediest patients, most of whom suffer various degrees of dementia (deteriorated mentality), including Alzheimer's disease. As a charge nurse, Harriette supervises a staff of four nurse assistants and is ultimately responsible for all the patients in her unit.

Harriette's day begins at 6:45 AM. Her first duty is to receive a fifteen-minute report from the outgoing charge nurse, who informs her of changes in a patient's condition or treatment occurring on her shift. Harriette then gathers together her crew of nursing assistants and discusses their assignments and any follow-up instructions for particular patients.

More Lingo to Learn

Obstetrics: *The branch of medicine dealing with childbirth.*

Occupational health nurse: *A nurse working, usually on-site, in a workplace setting, providing nursing services to employees there.*

Outpatient: *A person who is not a patient at a hospital, but who visits a clinic or dispensary connected with it for diagnosis or treatment.*

Pediatrics: *The branch of medicine dealing with the development, care, and diseases of children.*

Physiology: *The science dealing with the study of the function of tissues or organs.*

Psychiatric nursing: *A nursing specialty that deals with psychiatry; that is, mental, emotional, or behavioral disorders in patients.*

Public health nurse: *A nurse working for a community or government health organization stressing preventive medicine and social science.*

It is then time to begin AM care, which involves having the nursing assistants help their patients prepare for breakfast and for the day. They perform such basic duties as mouth care, bed baths, or assisting with clothes or showers. Harriette may monitor the group breakfast in the facility's cafeteria, surveying patients and talking to the nurse assistants seated among them about particular concerns. During this time, Harriette will also dispense medications ("pass meds") to those too infirm to eat in the cafeteria. She makes patient rounds and follows up on any required course of treatment. Because a patient fell the night before, Harriette must make sure that an X ray of the patient's fractured hip arrives from Radiology for the doctor to review. She will conduct such routine duties as calling patients' family members to update them, making doctor's appointments for patients, and monitoring those patients undergoing special medical procedures. She will insert and check catheters, feeding tubes, IVs, and so on, and make sure they are functioning properly. She will ensure that particular treatments are performed for patients with decubitus ulcers (bedsores) or pain control regimes. Special treatments might include turning patients over at scheduled times, applying dressings, or monitoring drugs dispensed via catheter and CAD pump. Although Harriette performs a large share of hands-on care, her primary role as charge nurse is one of quality control.

At 10:00 AM, the doctor arrives to perform rounds and Harriette gives him a status report. She accompanies the doctor through the unit, recording his orders in a "Doctor's Book." Perhaps a patient history or physical is due. The Doctor's Book serves as a communication tool, used by all medical staff on the unit to keep a running log of patient performance. It represents just one of several types of documentation that must be updated continually. Doctor's orders are recorded on "Physician Order Sheets" kept in the patient's chart, along with routine patient information, such as vital signs or physical therapy schedules. "Communication skills are primary," Harriette notes. "A licensed practical nurse or anyone working on the floor with patients must possess good verbal and written skills, because there is so much communication that takes place verbally and in writing with family members, doctors, other medical staff, and with the patients themselves."

//It is our job to take care of [the patients] and make them as comfortable as possible until their time comes. You get real close."

At 11:45 AM, the lunch trays come down, and the staff prepares to usher patients back to the cafeteria to assist them with their meals. Again, Harriette uses this opportunity to monitor her patients and staff. Did the nurse assistants fulfill all the needs of her patients? Did anything happen that she should be aware of? If it is not a doctor day, Harriette will assist with the feeding of patients and will interact with them and the nurse assistants. She will also start dispensing the "afternoon meds," after which she takes her own thirty-minute lunch break.

Harriette makes her last rounds from 2:00 to 2:30 PM and completes her daily charting, recording updated information on patients' charts and following up on anything noted during the previous twenty-four hours. She finalizes her shift and prepares to give turnover to the charge nurse coming in to relieve her at 2:45 PM. They confer and Harriette goes home, physically and sometimes mentally exhausted. Yet, she loves this job. "I love geriatrics," she says. "Maybe it's because I nursed my ailing aunt as a child, and because I lost my own moth-

WHAT IS IT LIKE TO BE A . . . ? CONTINUED

er when she was just forty-six years old. I often think of her when I'm working and wish she were here so I could take care of her."

Harriette can attest to the need for physical stamina in her job, as licensed practical nurses spend much of the working day on their feet, performing tasks that can be strenuous. The bedside care licensed practical nurses provide—helping patients bathe, sit up, get out of bed, stand, or walk—requires a fair share of reaching, bending, and stretching, which can sometimes subject them to back injuries. Most licensed practical nurses working in nursing homes or hospitals work a forty-hour week on a variety of shifts, including nights, weekends, and holidays. Licensed practical nurses working as private duty nurses can usually set their own work hours.

Along with the many rewards that licensed practical nurses experience in helping patients and medical staff with their care, some professional hazards do exist that include both physical and psychological stresses. As Harriette noted, the hands-on care that licensed practical nurses provide brings them very close to their patients, many of whom are very sick, in pain, or dying. They must sometimes deal with the demands of patients who are confused, agitated, or uncooperative. In addition to the emotional stress this close contact may bring, licensed practical nurses, particularly in hospitals, must also be mindful of potential exposure to caustic chemicals, radiation, and infectious diseases such as AIDS and hepatitis. Licensed practical nurses who provide in-home services often work long days and have a long adjustment period when moving to different homes to work with different patients, as each move requires adapting to new surroundings, patients, families, and physicians.

HAVE I GOT WHAT IT TAKES TO BE AN LPN?

"People should not enter this field thinking it's just a job," advises Norma Locke, a former licensed practical nurse who now works as a registered nurse in a suburban hospital outside of Washington, DC. "You have to love this job to do it well," she says. And that means having a natural longing to care for people. Like Harriette, Norma knew she wanted to be a nurse from the time she was a child and would plaster her dolls with Band-Aids and make tiny splints for their limbs.

Licensed practical nurses—and virtually anyone opting for a career in patient care—should also possess physical and mental stamina, patience, and endurance. John Word, executive director of the National Association for Practical Nurse Education and Service (NAPNES) and a former licensed practi-

To be a successful licensed practical nurse, you should:

Be mature, alert, and tactful, displaying patience and emotional stability

Maintain an objective point of view

Be able to follow detailed instructions and take correct action, particularly in a crisis

Have a caring, sympathetic nature and the flexibility to adapt to diverse situations

Possess good communication skills and the ability to assume responsibility

Be in good health and have physical stamina

cal nurse, cautions that while licensed practical nurses should possess a compassionate nature, they sometimes need to be thick-skinned when it comes to occasional unkind treatment from others. Doctors, nurses, and others who supervise licensed practical nurses, particularly in a hospital setting, are often under a lot of pressure and may take their frustrations out on those standing shoulder to shoulder with them in providing patient care. "Don't take it personally," he advises. As a licensed practical nurse, he never applied the self-label of "maid-servant," which he has heard some licensed practical nurses use to describe their perceived relationships to doctors. Norma, now a registered nurse, confided that as a licensed practical nurse in an acute care setting, she did sometimes feel like part of an underclass of health care providers, perceived by patients and co-workers alike as residing at the bottom of the totem pole. She admits that one of the reasons she went on to become a registered nurse was to upgrade her status and receive better treatment and more respect from patients and fellow workers.

In any case, all would agree that focusing on the higher goal of contributing to the health and well-being of people can counter the stresses of being on your feet all day or receiving unkind remarks from anguished patients or overburdened and frustrated doctors or supervisors. These qualities, along with good communication skills and the ability to follow directions, will help licensed practical nurses achieve a workable balance in their chosen field.

HOW DO I BECOME A LICENSED PRACTICAL NURSE?

EDUCATION

High School

To become a licensed practical nurse, you must first complete an approved practical nursing program in your state. Nearly all states require a high school degree to enroll in the program. Several states in the country, however, require that applicants complete only one or two years of high school. And some high schools even offer a practical nursing program that is approved by a state board of nursing or other regulatory body.

     Generally, if you have a broad educational background and wide-ranging interests you'll be prepared for the academic work and clinical practice required for the licensed practical nurse training program. Although many practical nursing schools do not require specific high school courses for admission, course offerings in science and mathematics—especially biology, chemistry, and physics—will give you a leg up when it comes time to start your advanced training. Because communication skills are critical to effective nursing, English and speech courses are also a good idea. But perhaps most importantly, you will need to have a caring, sympathetic nature, a sincere desire to contribute to the health and well-being of people, and the ability to follow oral and written directions.

Postsecondary Training

To be eligible to take the examination required for licensing, you must graduate from an approved school of practical nursing. (A correspondence course in practical nursing does not qualify you to take the state licensing examination.) The length of this program varies from state to state, depending on the individual state's admission requirements. Most programs last twelve months, although some are as long as eighteen months, and a few are less than a year. The trend now is toward an eighteen-month or two-year program leading to an associate's degree. The trend of expanded education speaks to the growing need for all nurses to have a broader base of knowledge. More complex technologies and the desire to minimize liability risks are reasons why. In fact, according to John Word, the American Nurses Association is trying to change the requirements for nurses to include a four-year bachelor's degree. Many nursing students, too, are opting for a four-year degree because of the accompanying increase in job status and opportunities.

     Licensed practical nurse programs are generally offered through two-year colleges and vocational and technical schools. Some programs are offered in high schools, hospitals, and colleges and universities. You must be eighteen years of age or older to apply; some programs actually have an upper age limit. Once enrolled, you will attend school five days a week, for six to eight hours a day. Participation in a practical nursing program is a full-time commitment. If you must work a part-time job while enrolled, be sure to consult the program director in advance to work out an arrangement. According to Harriette and other former practical nursing students, the program involves a lot of studying, referencing of notes, and staying in touch (after you finish the program) with professional resources.

Although practical nursing programs are no longer strictly hospital-based and contain more theory than clinical practice, they are generally affiliated with a hospital and include a clinical rotation along with classroom instruction. Classroom study covers basic nursing concepts, anatomy, physiology, medical-surgical nursing, pediatrics, obstetrics, psychiatric nursing, administration of drugs, nutrition, and first aid. Clinical practice usually takes place in a supervised hospital setting, but may include other settings as well. Students practice nursing techniques on mannequins before moving on to human patients. After successfully completing the program, students receive a diploma or certificate and may then take the state board licensing exam in the state where they plan to work.

Some schools have waiting lists for their practical nursing education programs. It is wise to plan early by obtaining and completing all application forms and beginning this process approximately one year ahead of intended enrollment. Contact several schools in your desired area and ask for their brochures, financial aid information, and application forms. Make sure the practical nursing program you select is approved by your state's board of nursing.

CERTIFICATION OR LICENSING

After graduating from an approved school of practical nursing, you will need to pass an examination to become licensed. All states and the District of Columbia require practical nurses to be licensed and to renew that license every two years. The state board of nursing issues the practical nursing license (or the vocational nursing license in California and Texas) once the National Council Licensure Examination for Practical Nurses, a written exam, is passed. Legal minimum requirements for the license are set by each state through its board of nursing, so these may vary from state to state. Licensed practical nurses in one state wishing to practice nursing in another state must apply to the board of nursing in that state. Although requirements vary slightly, it is generally not difficult to obtain another license and may not even require a written examination. Licensed practical nurses can identify themselves by putting the initials "LPN" or "LVN" (in Texas and California) after their names.

HOW DO I BECOME A . . . ?, CONTINUED

LABOR UNIONS

Although hospitals often have unions that medical employees are eligible to join, John Word advises against it. "Unions must be responsive to that block of their membership that is the strongest," he says, "and usually it is not the nurses." Rather, hospital unions often group professional employees with other employee groups whose interests do not converge with those of professional nurses. Consequently, union membership does not benefit those without the greatest voice within the membership. In the case where a union is formed only of nurses, at the same level, more benefits could be extracted, e.g., a union of practical nurses. He suggests, instead, membership with a professional association that has the interests and issues of the licensed practical nurse at its core as being far more beneficial.

WHO WILL HIRE ME?

John Word graduated from practical nursing school and received his license in 1955. He then secured a job at the hospital where he had been an orderly. New licensed practical nurses frequently step into part-time or full-time jobs with the hospitals where they did their training. Networking with staff may also uncover other job leads worth exploring. Harriette started her nursing career as a nurse assistant, but with encouragement from her supervisors at The Washington House, eventually enrolled in an eighteen-month practical nursing education program and earned her license. She acquired additional practical training at a Veterans Administration hospital, which, she says, allowed nurse assistants and licensed practical nurses greater involvement in learning and performing technical procedures on patients.

While veterans hospitals still employ a large number of licensed practical nurses, continued growth for licensed practical nurses working in hospitals generally is not expected to continue. This is due largely to the decreasing number of inpatients, which is related to cost concerns: it has become too costly for hospitals to care for patients for a prolonged recovery period.

Although the latest available statistics show the major employer of practical nurses still to be hospitals (40 percent), nursing homes are projected to take the lead in this regard, if they have not already. Nursing homes will offer the most new jobs for licensed practical nurses as the number of aged and disabled persons in need of long-term care rises rapidly with the aging "baby-boomer" population. Nursing homes will also be called on to care for the increasing number of convalescing patients who have been released from hospitals but are not recovered enough to go home.

There are many ways to find a job in this field. You may consider trying local employment agencies, although newspaper want ads may be the best avenue. Openings for licensed practical nurses are usually advertised in the classified section of the paper under headings such as "Nurses," "Licensed Practical Nurses," "LPNs," "Health Care," "Hospitals," "Private Duty," or "Temporary Nursing." You can also apply directly to hospitals, public health agencies, or nursing homes. Targeting a major hospital with acute care facilities may offer greater growth potential, and veterans hospitals in particular use a large number of licensed practical nurses to meet their ongoing need for basic, hands-on patient care. Applicants can send their resumes, with a short cover letter, directly to the personnel directors of health care facilities. Nurses associations and professional journals sometimes offer job leads and should be contacted individually.

Rapid growth for licensed practical nurse employment is also expected in such residential care facilities as board and care homes and group homes for the mentally disabled. In-home health care will also have high demand. Those interested in private duty nursing may be able to sign up with a hospital registry or with a physician's office. Employment is projected to grow rapidly in physicians' offices and clinics as well, including HMOs. Again, newspaper want ads are a good place to begin the job search, along with employment agencies. Large cities generally have employment agencies that specialize in jobs in the health care industry.

Advancement Possibilities

Charge nurses *oversee a particular floor or unit of a hospital, nursing home, or other health care setting.*

Nurse anesthetists *administer an anesthetic agent to patients before and during surgery to desensitize them to pain. They also work with pain management and respiratory management of patients.*

Physician assistants *provide health care services to patients under the direction and responsibility of a physician and may perform comprehensive physical examinations, compile patient medical data, administer or order diagnostic tests, and interpret test results.*

Registered nurses *have received a bachelor's degree in nursing and have been licensed by a state authority after qualifying for registration.*

WHERE CAN I GO FROM HERE?

After becoming a licensed practical nurse, John Word advanced through several related fields, including serving as an orthopedic technician at the same hospital where he was employed as a licensed practical nurse. Becoming a specialized medical technician required additional training and allowed him to do

WHERE CAN I GO FROM HERE?, CONTINUED

more complex medical procedures, such as drawing blood, starting IVs, performing portable X rays, and applying casts and splints—procedures that, at that time, practical nurses were not allowed to perform. By remaining active in his local association, securing several appointments to its board of directors on a volunteer basis, and moving on to elected posts at the national level, Word was eventually elected as the executive director of NAPNES in 1988, the position he holds today.

It is still true that licensed practical nurses can advance to higher-paying careers as medical technicians and registered nurses, and many do. Forty percent, in fact, use their licensed practical nurse designation as a stepping stone to greater pay and more responsibilities. There are several ways for an licensed practical nurse to climb the ladder. One is to locate similar positions in larger or more prestigious facilities where higher salaries are offered. It is also possible, by accumulating experience, to obtain supervisory duties over nurse assistants and nurses aides, as Harriette has done. Another way to advance is to do as Norma did and complete the additional education (usually two years at a community college) necessary to become a registered nurse.

But regardless of specialty or career ambition, licensed practical nurses must keep their skills current; participation in ongoing self-education is critical to job performance and advancement. "The health care field is constantly evolving," notes Word, "and we as medical professionals must continually update our skills to stay abreast of innovation and perform our jobs effectively." Nearly all of the licensed practical nurse association literature echoes this advice.

Participating in continuing education courses is a good way to stay current with the technological advances and growing complexity of patient care techniques and procedures. Some states even require a minimum number of continuing education hours before they will renew the practical nursing license every two years. Continuing education programs may be sponsored by a variety of organizations, including community colleges, government agencies, vocational-technical institutes, private educational firms, and local, state, and national health associations. Licensed practical nurses must assess the educational opportunities available in their communities and determine which are the most relevant for maintaining their practice skills.

Another method of improving skills and growing in the field is to take advantage of in-service educational programs that more and more employers are offering. These may include seminars, workshops, and clinical sessions on relevant work topics. Taking advantage of these in-house opportunities will help the licensed practical nurse accumulate additional skills and may even lead to more specialized and higher-paying careers. Some hospitals offer programs that teach licensed practical nurses to do kidney dialysis or to work with patients in cardiac or intensive care units, which may lead to more specialized job titles.

John Word also strongly recommends reading the available literature to stay current. These publications will also keep the reader apprised of the most modern nursing textbooks, which he recommends over all the other literature for staying up-to-date in the nursing field.

WHAT ARE SOME RELATED JOBS?

The U.S. Department of Labor classifies licensed practical nurses under the headings "Occupations in Medicine and Health, Not Elsewhere Classified" and "Nursing." Also under this heading are people who work closely with patients to provide basic care; perform associated documentation tasks; assist other medical personnel before and during surgery; perform emergency medical care and interpret laboratory tests; and conduct patient examinations and document problems and progress.

Related Jobs

General duty nurses

In-service coordinators of auxiliary personnel

Medical assistants

Nurse anesthetists

Nurse-midwives

Nurse practitioners

Optometric assistants

Private duty nurses

Psychiatric technicians

Registered nurses

Veterinary technicians

WHAT ARE THE SALARY RANGES?

The salary range for licensed practical nurses varies considerably between geographic locations and between institutions, and depends on many factors, including experience and responsibilities. Median weekly earnings of full-time salaried LPNs were $468 in 1996. The top 10 percent earned more than $673 a week, the middle 50 percent earned between $388 and $563 a week, and the lowest 10 percent earned less than $318 a week.

Hospitals tend to pay a little more than nursing homes and long-term care centers. According to a University of Texas Medical Branch survey of hospitals and medical centers, the median salary of licensed practical nurses working full-time, excluding shift differentials, was $23,394 in 1994. And the Buck Survey, conducted by the American Health Care Association in 1996, found that licensed practical nurses in chain nursing homes had median

WHAT ARE THE SALARY RANGES?, CONTINUED

hourly earnings of $12.00 in 1996. The middle 50 percent earned between $10.60 and $13.50 an hour.

For accurate information on wage scales for licensed practical nurses in the community where you want to work, call a hospital in the area, ask for the personnel department, and inquire about salaries for newly licensed practical nurses. Other sources include registries, long-term care facilities, or the visiting nurse associations, which can provide specific details on licensed practical nurse wage scales.

Licensed practical nurses also usually receive fringe benefits, such as paid sick, holiday, and vacation time, medical coverage, 401 K plans, and other perks depending on the employer.

WHAT IS THE JOB OUTLOOK?

The job outlook is excellent for licensed practical nurses and everyone choosing a medical health care profession. As the number of students graduating from practical nursing schools continues to rise, so does the demand for their services. The general growth in health care and the long-term health care needs of an aging population help ensure the continued need for licensed practical nurses and other health care professionals over the next ten years. In fact, employment of licensed practical nurses is expected to increase faster than average for all occupations through the year 2006, in response to the needs of a rapidly growing older population and to the cost constraints hospitals experience relative to providing long-term patient care. As in most other occupations, replacement needs will be the main source of job openings.

As mentioned previously, most new jobs for licensed practical nurses will be in nursing homes and long-term care facilities that cater to the growing aging population. These agencies will also house recovering patients released from hospitals but not yet well enough to return home. State and federal regulations on nursing homes are requiring them to hire more licensed practical nurses in lieu of other so-called "health aides," who may be given minimal training, are unlicensed, and often under-qualified to administer patient care. A similar demand for licensed practical nurses will occur in physicians' offices and clinics, including HMOs, concerned with liability issues. New rules and regulations set out by insurance companies shortening the length of stay allowed for patients in a facility will create a great demand for private duty nurses. Rapid growth is expected in board and care homes and group homes for the mentally disabled as well.

Nurse Anesthetist

SUMMARY

DEFINITION
Nurse anesthetists *are registered nurses (RNs) with advanced education in anesthesiology. They are responsible for administering, supervising, and monitoring anesthesia-related care for patients undergoing surgical procedures.*

ALTERNATIVE JOB TITLE
Certified registered nurse anesthetist (CRNA)

SALARY RANGE
$60,000 to $73,444 to $100,000+

EDUCATIONAL REQUIREMENTS
Master's degree

CERTIFICATION OR LICENSING
All RNs are required to pass a licensing exam; an additional certification exam is mandatory for nurse anesthetists.

EMPLOYMENT OUTLOOK
Faster than the average

HIGH SCHOOL SUBJECTS
Biology
Chemistry
English (writing/literature)
Mathematics
Physics

PERSONAL INTERESTS
Helping people: emotionally
Helping people: physical health/medicine

"Good," Andy says, looking at the clock. "It's not yet 6:30 and I'm on schedule." Andy Griffin, a nurse anesthetist, has checked the anesthesia machine and made sure that the oxygen meter and monitoring devices are working properly. He has laid out the tubes and other essentials that will be used in the first operation of the day—the removal of a middle-aged man's diseased gall bladder.

Andy picks up the patient's chart and carefully reviews it. By 7 AM, he will be greeting the patient in the holding room to begin the process of administering general anesthesia.

WHAT DOES A NURSE ANESTHETIST DO?

Nurse anesthetists, also known as certified registered nurse anesthetists (CRNAs), are registered nurses with advanced training in anesthesiology. Reliable methods of putting a patient to sleep were first developed in the 1840s when the discovery of ether anesthesia revolutionized surgery. Before that time, when surgery offered the only possible chance of saving a person's life (if a gangrenous leg had to be amputated, for example), all that the surgeon could

WHAT DOES A NURSE ANESTHETIST DO?, CONTINUED

do was to offer alcohol or opium to deaden the pain and then saw off the limb as quickly as possible before the patient went into shock.

Anesthesiologists are physicians who completed a residency in anesthesiology and passed medical board exams in that specialty. Before World War II, only seven anesthesiology physician residency programs were available; in 1942, there were seventeen nurse anesthetists for every anesthesiologist. During the first half of the century, medical students and physicians were often trained by nurse anesthetists in anesthesiology techniques.

Approximately 26 million anesthetic procedures are carried out annually in U.S. medical facilities; more than 65 percent of these are administered by nurse anesthetists. In 85 percent of rural hospitals, nurse anesthetists are the only anesthesia providers.

Contemporary anesthesiology is far more complicated than in the early days when an ether- or chloroform-soaked cloth or sponge was held up to the patient's face. In advance of surgery, a nurse anesthetist takes the patient's history, evaluates his or her anesthesia needs, and forms a plan for the best possible management of the case (often in consultation with an anesthesiologist). The nurse anesthetist also explains the planned procedures to the patient and answers questions. On the morning of the operation, the nurse anesthetist administers an intravenous (IV) sedative to relax the patient.

Usually a combination of several anesthetic agents is administered by the nurse anesthetist to establish and maintain the patient in a controlled state of unconsciousness, insensibility to pain, and muscular relaxation. Muscular relaxant drugs prevent the transmission of nerve impulses to the muscles to ensure that involuntary movements by the unconscious patient will not interfere with the surgery. Some general anesthetics are administered by inhalation through a mask and tube— the most common are nitrous oxide,

Lingo to Learn

Analgesic: *Pain-relieving medication.*

Epidural: *Local anesthesia administered by injection into the space just outside the dural sac that surrounds the spinal cord.*

Holding room: *Room just outside the operating room where the patient is prepared for surgery.*

Infiltration: *Local anesthesia administered by injection directly into the surgical area.*

IV, Intravenous: *Refers to anesthetics or any other substance administered through a vein.*

Nerve block: *Local anesthesia administered by injection near the nerves that control sensation in the surgical area.*

Spinal: *Local anesthesia administered by injection into the dural sac that surrounds the spinal cord, resulting in loss of sensation in the entire body below that point in the spinal cord.*

Tertiary health care: *The high-tech specialized diagnosis and treatment available only at large research and teaching hospitals.*

Topical: *Local anesthesia administered by applying a drug to the surface of a mucous membrane that absorbs it; a method often used for surgery on the eye, nose, or throat.*

halothane, enflurane, and isoflurane. Others are administered intravenously. Because the muscular relaxants prevent patients from breathing on their own, the nurse anesthetist has to provide artificial respiration through a tube inserted into the windpipe.

Throughout the surgery, the nurse anesthetist monitors the patient's vital signs (blood pressure, respiration, heart rate, and temperature) by watching the video and digital displays. The nurse anesthetist is also responsible for maintaining the patient's blood, water, and salt levels and—from moment to moment—readjusting the flow of anesthetics and other medications to ensure optimal results. After surgery, nurse anesthetists monitor their patients' return to consciousness and watch for complications; they may also be involved in postoperative pain management.

General anesthesia is not necessary for all surgical procedures. Nurse anesthetists also work on cases in which they provide various types of local anesthesia—topical, infiltration, nerve—block, spinal, and epidural or caudal.

WHAT IS IT LIKE TO BE A NURSE ANESTHETIST?

Andy Griffin sometimes tells people that the existence of the nurse anesthetist is "one of the best-kept secrets in the United States." He discovered nurse anesthetists during a summer job as an operating room assistant (orderly) during his undergraduate days. Andy already knew he was interested in pursuing a career in the medical field, and watching the work of nurse anesthetists in the operating room made him recognize what a challenging job that would be.

After receiving his bachelor's degree in nursing and becoming a licensed RN, Andy worked for two years in a hospital intensive care unit (ICU) before beginning a master's degree program in anesthesiology. Although he is still a few months away from graduation at the Middle Tennessee School of Anesthesia, he has already worked as nurse anesthetist on nearly seven hundred cases. After graduation, he will be working for an anesthesia group that has contracts with three Nashville hospitals—St. Thomas, Baptist, and Centennial.

Today would be fairly typical, thought Andy. After the 7:30 AM gall bladder, there would be several other surgical patients. Occasionally, one complicated operation would take all day; recently he was on an open-heart operation that lasted from 7:30 AM to 3:00 PM.

It might be a typical day, but there are never any merely "routine" cases. At every moment of the surgery, Andy has to be vigilant—watching the dials on the equipment, adjusting the levels of anesthetic agents being administered (some phases of the operation required deeper anesthesia than others), and monitoring the patient's respiration. During the first month or so of his master's program, Andy had learned the basic facts of anesthesia—the various anesthetic agents available and how to calculate dosage on the basis of the patient's weight. The next two years were spent learning how to anticipate problems; he had to learn what to do in the 5 percent of cases that do not go as planned.

Sometimes, for example, it turns out to be impossible to maintain an airway without performing a tracheotomy (an incision in the throat to insert a breathing tube into the windpipe, or trachea). "The surgeon stays with the surgery," Andy explained. "Life support is the nurse anesthetist's responsibility." At the hospitals where Andy works, an anesthesiologist who is responsible for monitoring four to six operating rooms at the same time is available for consultation in a crisis.

As the surgeon begins closing the incision, Andy simultaneously reduces the anesthesia in order to bring the patient back to consciousness. After the surgery, Andy pulls out the breathing tube as soon as the patient is alert enough to respond to his or her name. When patients are stable, which usually means awake and breathing independently, Andy turns them over to the recovery room nurse.

Carole Rietz is a nurse anesthetist and clinical nurse specialist in Vanderbilt University Hospital's pediatrics division. She works with children and adolescents; her patients range in age from premature infants to eighteen-year-olds. She occasionally has patients over the age of eighteen whose special needs make it most appropriate for them to be treated in pediatrics.

Since Carole shares responsibility with anesthesiologists for the care of her patients before, during, and after surgery, she must be skilled in the use of

In-depth

The first nurse anesthetist was Sister Mary Bernard, who practiced in Pennsylvania in the 1870s. The first school of nurse anesthetists was founded in 1909 at St. Vincent Hospital in Portland, Oregon. Since then, many schools have been established, including the famous Mayo Clinic Anesthesia Program.

During World War I, America's nurse anesthetists were the major providers of care to the troops in France. They also trained the French and British nurses and physicians in anesthesia procedures.

Prior to World War II, anesthesia was considered a nursing specialty. In 1942, there were seventeen nurse anesthetists in the United States for every anesthesiologist.

The nurse anesthesia specialty was formally created on June 17, 1931, when the American Association of Nurse Anesthetists (AANA) held its first meeting.

FYI

Approximately 26 million anesthetic procedures are carried out annually in U.S. medical facilities— and more than 65 percent of these are administered by nurse anesthetists. In 85 percent of rural hospitals, nurse anesthetists are the only anesthesia providers.

airways, ventilators, IVs, blood- and fluid-replacement techniques, and postoperative pain management.

Some children come to the hospital for one-time operations, such as a tonsillectomy, appendectomy, or hernia repair. Those with long-term medical problems may need to return for surgery and/or other treatment on a regular basis. Many of Carole's patients are children with serious chronic illnesses; some are premature infants with complicated health problems requiring a series of surgeries. Carole works closely with physicians in various pediatric subspecialties (anesthesiology, oncology, orthopedics, urology, and others) and with clinical nurse specialists to ensure the best possible care for each child.

Communicating with children and their parents is an important part of Carole's job. Providing the best possible physical care for patients is obviously essential, yet psychological and social needs are also vital. Vanderbilt tries to provide a nonthreatening hospital environment with approachable staff members. Children and parents can take tours of the facility, where the equipment and medical procedures being planned for the child are explained. Parents need to be trained as primary caregivers in the home, especially in cases of long-term health problems. "If the mother is comfortable, then that feeling of confidence is transferred to the child," explains Carole.

It is essential to answer children's questions at the appropriate age level. A four-year-old with cancer or failing kidneys is still a four-year-old with a child's perspective. Caregivers need to be constantly aware that children do not think like adults.

Carole stresses the importance of giving children choices, whenever possible, to help them feel that they have some say in what is happening to them. They may choose a breathing mask in one of several flavors, or they may bring a favorite toy with them into the operating room. If the child will be returning frequently to the hospital, Carole tries to arrange for care from the same providers each time to avoid the anxiety of having to meet new staff members on every visit.

Carole especially appreciates the team-oriented, problem-solving approach to health care. After more than thirty years in nursing, Carole strongly believes that health care providers must take an active role in fighting for their patients to prevent the "business perspective" from taking over medicine.

HAVE I GOT WHAT IT TAKES TO BE A NURSE ANESTHETIST?

Nurse anesthetists must be able to concentrate intently for lengthy periods. They are responsible for keeping the anesthetized patient alive, which requires careful attention to every detail. They need to be critical thinkers who can analyze problems accurately and swiftly, make decisions, and take appropriate action. All nurses need the ability to remain calm during emergencies; the operating room is one of the most stressful environments around.

To be a successful nurse anesthetist, you should:

Be able to analyze and solve problems quickly

Be able to handle stressful situations

Be able to remain calm in emergencies

Have strong powers of concentration

Research studies of anesthesia-related problems have demonstrated that most could have been avoided if the anesthesia provider had monitored the patient's condition more vigilantly. The Journal of the American Medical Association published guidelines called the Harvard Minimal Monitoring Standards on Anesthesia Care in 1986. More recently, the American Association of Nurse Anesthetists issued even more detailed monitoring standards.

Nurse anesthetists also need to be efficient in their time management. "The surgeons have to be kept happy by having the patients moved along quickly without long delays between cases," said one nurse anesthetist put it. If a nurse anesthetist is slow in finishing one case and setting up for the next, the surgeon may be reluctant to work with that individual again.

HOW DO I BECOME A NURSE ANESTHETIST?

EDUCATION

High School

To become a nurse anesthetist, you must first be a registered nurse. Anyone who is interested in a nursing career needs to take a college-preparatory course in high school that gives a good foundation in the laboratory sciences. You need to take biology, chemistry, physics, and mathematics. If your high school offers advanced biology or a human physiology course beyond the introductory biology class, these would be good choices for electives. English classes and other courses that develop communication skills are also important.

High school would be a good time to test your interest in nursing by getting some hands-on experience. There may be opportunities for volunteer work or a part-time job at a hospital, community health center, or nursing

Q. What's New in Learning?
A. Preceptorships

A preceptorship is really a new and improved version of shadowing. You know shadowing, like when you go to work with your mom or dad and follow them around to see what they do on the job. Preceptorships take shadowing a huge step forward and they are really something to look into. A preceptorship is an arrangement where a student (that would be you) is assigned on a one-to-one basis to a clinical nurse expert in a certain area. What's innovative about this method is that you are not only learning what someone else does as a nurse, you are learning how you will react and respond to nursing. That's a whole new ball game! Basically, this year-long adventure in nursing is the best hands-on class you can have, with your very own expert to make sure you know what you're doing. Look into this type of opportunity when you're starting an entry level job or looking for supplementary learning.

home in your community. You might also talk with people in various nursing fields or join a Future Nurses Club.

Postsecondary Training

There are three ways to become a registered nurse—a two-year associate's degree program at a junior or community college, a three-year hospital nursing school program, or a bachelor's degree program (BSN) at a college or university nursing school. Sometimes persons who already have a bachelor's degree in another field enter nursing through a master's-level program (MSN) rather than by earning another bachelor's degree. All programs combine classroom education and actual nursing experience. Part-time or summer jobs in health care offer additional opportunities for exploring the nursing field.

The bachelor's or master's degree route is strongly recommended since a nurse with less than a BSN has few opportunities for advancement. All applicants to nurse anesthetist programs are required to have at least a bachelor's degree. (The other advanced-practice nursing fields—nurse practitioner, clinical nurse specialist, and nurse midwife—also expect applicants to have a bachelor's degree before beginning specialized training.)

Undergraduate nursing programs include courses in biology, microbiology, human anatomy and physiology, psychology, nutrition, and statistics. Some classes in humanities and social sciences are also required in BSN programs. After completing the nursing degree, it is necessary to pass a national licensing exam; only then are you a registered nurse.

There are over ninety accredited nurse anesthesia programs in the United States. They last twenty-four to thirty-six months and nearly all offer a master's degree. There are also a few clinical nursing doctorate programs for nurse anesthetists. (Beginning in 1998, the few programs that were offering only a certificate in anesthesiology will be required to offer at least a master's degree.) Applicants to nurse anesthetist programs must have at least one year

HOW DO I BECOME A . . . ?, CONTINUED

of experience as an RN in an intensive care unit; many have considerably more. The admissions process is competitive. Andy Griffin recently estimated that the average undergraduate grade point average of the students at the Middle Tennessee School of Anesthesia was about a 3.5 on a 4.0 scale.

If you are enrolled in a nurse anesthetist program, expect to take classes in pharmacology (the science of drugs and their uses), anatomy and physiology, pathophysiology (the physiology of disease), biochemistry, chemistry, and physics. You'll also acquire hundreds of hours of anesthesia-related clinical experience in surgery and obstetrics.

CERTIFICATION OR LICENSING

Nurse anesthetists are required to pass national certification exams after completing their educational program. The certification process was initiated by the American Association of Nurse Anesthetists in 1945. All states recognize certified registered nurse anesthetist status. Nurse anesthetists are not required to work under the supervision of an anesthesiologist, although some licensing laws do stipulate that they must work with a physician.

WHO WILL HIRE ME?

Many nurse anesthetists are employed by hospitals or outpatient surgery centers (this would include dental and podiatry work as well as same-day surgery). Others are in group or independent practice and provide services to hospitals and other health care centers on a contract basis. Some work for the U.S. Public Health Services. Most rural hospitals rely on nurse anesthetists as their only providers of anesthesia. Nurse anesthetists are eligible to receive direct Medicare reimbursement (under the 1986 Omnibus Budget Reconciliation Act).

The U.S. military also employs nurse anesthetists. In every twentieth-century war, nurse anesthetists were the major providers of anesthesia care, especially in forward-positioned medical facilities. In the Vietnam War, there were three nurse anesthetists for every physician anesthetist.

FYI

For centuries, alcohol, opium, mandrake, hemp, and henbane were given orally or by inhalation during surgery or childbirth. The Indians of Peru chewed the leaves of the coca plant—from which cocaine is derived—and used their saliva to reduce local pain during surgery.

Because the high-quality, cost-effective anesthesia service provided by nurse anesthetists is widely acknowledged, more and more health care institutions are eager to employ them.

WHERE CAN I GO FROM HERE?

Experienced nurse anesthetists can earn over $100,000 a year. Those who want new professional challenges beyond direct practice might consider teaching or administrative positions or involvement in research for improved or specialized anesthesia equipment and procedures. Some nurse anesthetists choose to acquire other advanced-practice nursing qualifications so they can be involved in a wider range of nursing activities. Doctoral programs for nurse anesthetists are expected to expand in the near future.

WHAT ARE SOME RELATED JOBS?

The U.S. Department of Labor classifies nurse anesthetists with others in nursing occupations. Among these workers are nurse-midwives, private and general duty nurses, nurse practitioners, and school nurses. The U.S. Department of Labor also classifies nurse anesthetists with other registered nurses. Among these workers are office nurses, directors of nursing services, directors of schools of nursing, and community health nurses.

Related Jobs

Community health nurses

Directors of nursing services

Directors of schools of nursing

Nurse-midwives

Nurse practitioners

Office nurses

Private and general duty nurses

School nurses

WHAT ARE THE SALARY RANGES?

Nurse anesthetists are probably the highest paid nursing specialists. Salaries range from the $60,000s to the $80,000s to over $100,000 for experienced nurse anesthetists. According to the Hay Group's survey of acute care hospitals, the median annual base salary of full-time nurse anesthetists was $82,000 in January 1997. The middle 50 percent earned between $74,700 and $90,300. Anesthesiologists, by contrast, average over $220,000.

Nurse anesthetists also receive fringe benefits such as paid sick, holiday, and vacation time, medical coverage, 401-K plans, and other perks depending on the employer.

WHAT IS THE JOB OUTLOOK?

The job outlook for nurse anesthetists is excellent. Today, Certified Registered Nurse Anesthetists working with anesthesiologists, physicians, and, where authorized, podiatrists, dentists, and other health care providers, administer

WHAT IS THE JOB OUTLOOK?, CONTINUED

approximately 65 percent of all anesthetics given each year in the United States. CRNAs work in every setting in which anesthesia is delivered: tertiary care centers, community hospitals, labor and delivery rooms, ambulatory surgical centers, diagnostic suites, and physician offices. CRNAs are the sole anesthesia providers in more than 70 percent of rural hospitals, affording anesthesia and resuscitative services to these medical facilities for surgical, obstetrical, and trauma care. Furthermore, ten nurse anesthetists can be educated for the cost of educating one anesthesiologist. In addition to the much higher annual cost of educating an anesthesiology resident, the total educational process for producing a nurse anesthetist (including undergraduate and graduate work) is on average four years shorter. All of these factors combine to make the likelyhood for continued reliance on nurse anesthetists very good.

Nurse Assistant

SUMMARY

DEFINITION
Nurse assistants care for patients in hospitals and nursing homes under the supervision of nurses.

ALTERNATIVE JOB TITLES
Nurse or nursing aide
Nursing assistant
Orderly

SALARY RANGE
$13,000 to $14,612 to $25,000

EDUCATIONAL REQUIREMENTS
High school diploma; completion of training program in either a community college or vocational school

CERTIFICATION OR LICENSING
Voluntary for hospitals
Mandatory for nursing homes

EMPLOYMENT OUTLOOK
Faster than the average

HIGH SCHOOL SUBJECTS
Biology
English (writing/literature)
Health
Sociology

PERSONAL INTERESTS
Helping people: emotionally
Helping people: physical health/medicine

Hurrying about to answer call lights; helping nursing home residents get showered, dressed, and off to breakfast; taking residents to the bathroom—it had been a hectic morning and now Dorothy Reeve must make a bed. It may not seem like a large task, but the resident is bedridden and fragile and can't be moved about much. Dorothy will leave the resident in the bed while making it; she'll work slowly and carefully, a contrast from the fast action that's been required of her all morning.

First Dorothy draws the curtain to protect the resident's privacy. "Are you comfortable, Mrs. Lanning?" she asks, adjusting the pillow and raising the bed. When she's certain that the resident is at ease and unexposed, she lowers the side rail and begins to make up half the bed. She then raises the side rail again and helps the resident to the other side of the bed to finish. Before leaving, she checks again with Mrs. Lanning to make certain she's comfortable and has everything she needs. Mrs. Lanning responds with a smile and she squeezes Dorothy's hand. Dorothy leaves the room with the certainty that her tasks, though small and routine, are important to the residents and the home.

WHAT DOES A NURSE ASSISTANT DO?

Though the job title suggests someone who assists nurses, nurse assistants actually perform many duties independently; in some cases, they become more closely involved with patients or nursing home residents than do registered nurses. Nurse assistants work under the supervision of nurses and perform tasks that allow the nursing staff to perform their primary duties effectively and efficiently.

Nurse assistants perform basic nursing care in hospitals and nursing homes. Male nurse assistants are perhaps better known as orderlies. Working independently and alongside nurses and doctors, nurse assistants help move patients, assist in patients' exercise and nutrition, and see to the patients' personal hygiene. They bring the patients their meal trays and help them to eat. They push the patients on stretchers and in wheelchairs to operating and X-ray rooms. They also help to admit and discharge patients. Nurse assistants must keep charts of their work for review by nurses.

About half of the nurse assistants today work in nursing homes, tending to the daily care of elderly residents. They help residents with baths and showers, meals, and exercise. They help them in and out of their beds and to and from the bathroom. They also record the health of residents by taking body temperatures and checking blood pressures.

Because the residents are living within such close proximity to each other, and because they need help with personal hygiene and health care, a nurse assistant also takes care to protect the privacy of the resident. It is the responsibility of a nurse assistant to make the resident feel as comfortable as possible. Nurse assistants may also work with patients who are not fully functional, teaching them how to care for themselves, educating them in personal hygiene and health care.

The work can be strenuous, requiring the lifting and moving of patients. Nurse assistants must work with partners, or in groups, when performing the more strenuous tasks, so that neither the nurse assistant nor the resident is injured. Some requirements of the job can be as routine as changing sheets and helping a resident with phone calls, while other requirements can be as difficult and unattractive as assisting a resident with elimination and cleaning up a resident who has vomited.

Lingo to Learn

Ambulatory care: *Serving patients who are able to walk.*

Acute care: *Providing emergency services and general medical and surgical treatment for acute disorders rather than long-term care.*

Asepsis: *Methods of sterilization to ensure the absence of germs.*

Gerontology: *A branch of medicine that deals with aging and the problems of the aged.*

Neonatal: *Pertaining to newborn children.*

Pediatrics: *A branch of medicine concerned with the development, care, and diseases of babies and children.*

FYI

There are about 1.4 million nurse assistants in the country; half are employed in nursing homes.

Nurse assistants may be called upon by nurses and physicians to perform the more menial and unappealing tasks, but they also have the opportunity to develop meaningful relationships with residents. Nurse assistants work closely with residents, often gaining their trust and admiration. When residents are having personal problems, or problems with the staff, they may turn to the nurse assistant for help.

Nurse assistants generally work a forty-hour workweek, with some overtime. The hours and weekly schedule may be irregular, however, depending on the needs of the care institution. An assistant may have one day off in the middle of the week, followed by three days of work, then another day off. Nurse assistants are needed around the clock, so beginning assistants may be required to work late at night or very early in the morning.

WHAT IS IT LIKE TO BE A NURSE ASSISTANT?

Dorothy Reeve works in the Medicare wing of a ninety-resident nursing home in Petaluma, California. "I clock in at 7:00 AM," she says, "and I hit the floor." She works under the supervision of registered nurses and LVNs (licensed vocational nurses), as well as therapists (physical, occupational, and speech). But mostly she performs her own set of daily responsibilities. Dorothy starts by getting three or four residents out of bed and helps them to start their day. Getting a patient out of bed sometimes requires a mechanical lift. "The lift," Dorothy explains, "supports their weight under a sling and they are lifted like an engine from a car." Also, Dorothy works with another nurse assistant who helps with lifting and feeding. "There are twenty-one residents on our wing when full," she says. By taking turns with a partner each nurse assistant can take breaks as well as keep watch over residents in the wing.

"I give the person a shower if it's scheduled," she says, "and I get them dressed if they are unable to dress themselves." The residents have set schedules and many must be up at certain times for physical therapy and other appointments. Once her residents are dressed, they are brought out to the dining hall for breakfast. Breakfast is served from 8:00 AM until around 9:00 AM.

"We have to be done with our morning care by 11:00 AM," she says. In addition to getting patients ready for the day, Dorothy must attend to call lights; call lights are the way residents signal the nurse assistants for help. "You have to make sure that the call lights are answered within three minutes," Dorothy says. "It's the law." Call lights usually have accompanying noises to alert the assistant. "You have to constantly be aware of the sounds that are normal and be alert for the sounds that are not." The call lights typically go off throughout the morning, and through breakfast and lunch.

Dorothy also takes the residents' vital signs and reports any abnormal readings. She says, "You really have to know your residents individually to know if they're feeling up to par."

When caring for a resident, privacy is important. "We have to make sure that when the residents are receiving personal care," Dorothy says, "that the privacy curtains are pulled and no one can see in. We make sure the door is firmly shut and the drapes are pulled closed for the resident's dignity."

> **"You really have to know your residents individually to know if they're feeling up to par."**

After helping patients with their morning routines and appointments, then helping them with their lunch, Dorothy takes some of the residents to the bathroom and helps them lay down for a rest. "Then I get all my information together for legal charting," she says. "The charts we keep are legal documents and when we sign our name we are liable for all the information we chart. If there are any legal questions at sometime in the future we had better know why we charted what we did. The state inspectors look at our charting and the RNs get a lot of their information from our viewpoint and from what we chart." Dorothy spends thirty minutes or more preparing the day's chart. To assist in chart preparation, she records her work throughout the day so she doesn't have to try to remember everything she did for each individual resident.

Dorothy's day is usually complete at 3:00 PM, though she occasionally works overtime. She is paid for 37.5 hours a week and works a rotating schedule; this means she works three to four days, then has two days off, and then starts the cycle again.

HAVE I GOT WHAT IT TAKES TO BE A NURSE ASSISTANT?

A nurse assistant must care about the work and the patients and must show a general understanding and compassion for the ill, disabled, and the elderly. Because of the rigorous physical demands placed on a nurse assistant, you

To be a successful nurse assistant, you should:

Be a compassionate person

Be in good health

Be able to perform some heavy lifting

Have a great deal of patience

Take orders well

Be a good team player

Be emotionally stable

should be in good health. Also, the hours and responsibilities of the job won't allow you to take many sick days. Along with this good physical health, you should have good mental health, as well. The job can be emotionally demanding, requiring your patience and stability. You should also be able to take orders and to work as part of a team.

Though the work can often be rewarding, a nurse assistant must also be prepared for the worst. "When I first started," Dorothy says, "I had the illusion that the patients would be just like my grandmother was at the time—baking, sewing, alert." But she almost quit after the first week. "The residents hit, they screamed, they fell down. You had to feed them their meals and they could not shower themselves." But, after her training, Dorothy came to appreciate the work and to care about the residents. "I like people," she says, "and I love to take care of them. I like to see them smile. In some cases, we care givers are the only family they have now." Dorothy also appreciates the steadiness of the work and the certainty that experienced nurse assistants will always be in high demand.

How Do I Become a Nurse Assistant?

Dorothy has worked in nursing homes for more than thirteen years. She completed high school and has earned some junior college credits. She has also completed a state-required training program and received certification. Dorothy found the training process to be overwhelming at first. "There's so much to remember," she says. "And you need to learn everything quickly so that you can work on your own."

EDUCATION

High School

Communication skills are valuable for a nurse assistant, so take English, speech, and writing courses. Science courses, such as biology and anatomy, will also prepare you for future training. Because a high school diploma is not required of nurse assistants, many high school students are hired by nursing homes and hospitals for part-time work. Job opportunities may also exist in a hospital or nursing home kitchen, introducing you to diet and nutrition. Also, volunteer work can familiarize you with the work nurses and nurse assistants perform, as well as introduce you to some medical terminology.

Postsecondary Training

Nurse assistants are not required to have a college degree but may have to complete a short training course at a community college or vocational school. These training courses, usually instructed by a registered nurse, teach basic nursing skills and prepare students for the state certification exam. Nurse assistants typically begin the training courses after getting their first job as an assistant, and the course work is incorporated into their on-the-job training.

Many people work as nurse assistants as they pursue other medical professions; someone interested in becoming a nurse or a paramedic may work as an assistant while taking courses. A high school student or a student in a premedical program may work as a nurse assistant part-time before going on to medical school.

CERTIFICATION OR LICENSING

Nurse assistants in hospitals are not required to be certified but those working in nursing homes must pass a state exam. The Omnibus Budget Reconciliation Act (OBRA) passed by Congress in 1987 requires nursing homes to hire only certified nurse assistants.

Dorothy says, "Certification took almost six months of training and class work. California has very strict guidelines." OBRA also requires continuing education for nurse assistants, and periodic evaluations.

WHO WILL HIRE ME?

One-half of all nurse assistants work in nursing homes. Other places where they are employed include hospitals, halfway houses, retirement centers, and private homes. Dorothy started working as a nurse assistant when she was twenty-one years old. "I had two children to support," she says, "and this field has always interested me because I've always liked older people. And they offered to pay me as I learned." Dorothy heard about the job through a friend and visited the nursing facility directly and filled out an application. She began training in 1984; she worked for the same nursing facility for a year, then worked in a few other homes in the area over the following few years. She then returned to the place where she trained and has stayed there for nine years. It is typical for nurse assistants to try different facilities after receiving training.

Because of the high demand for nurse assistants, you can apply directly to the health care facilities in your area. Most will probably have a human resources department that advertises positions in the newspaper and interviews applicants.

WHERE CAN I GO FROM HERE?

One of the things Dorothy appreciates about her work is that it allows her to perform many of the tasks and duties of a nurse. "Some day I would like to get my nursing degree," she says. But she emphasizes that she is very happy in her current position. "I would like the extra training, but I don't want to just push pills and sit behind a desk and not get to know the residents like I do now." Dorothy would also be interested in trying her work in a different setting, like a hospital.

For the most part, there is not much opportunity for advancement within the job of nurse assistant. To move up in a health care facility requires additional training. Some nurse assistants, after gaining experience and learning medical technology, enroll in nursing programs, or may even decide to pursue medical degrees.

Related Jobs

Ambulance attendants

Child care attendants

Emergency medical technicians

Home health aides

Morgue attendants

Occupational therapy aides

Optometric assistants

Orderlies

Perfusionists

Physical therapy aides

Psychiatric aides

Surgical technicians

A nursing home requires a lot of hard work and dedication so nurse assistants frequently burnout, or quit before completing their training. Others may choose another aspect of the job, such as working as a home health aide. Helping patients in their homes, these aides see to the client's personal health, hygiene, and home care.

WHAT ARE SOME RELATED JOBS?

The U.S. Department of Labor classifies nurse assistants with workers in patient care. Included in this group are home health aides, occupational therapy aides, ambulance attendants, emergency medical technicians, orderlies, perfusionists, psychiatric

What Are the Related Jobs?, continued

aides, surgical technicians, and optometric assistants. The U.S. Department of Labor also classifies nurse assistants with attendants in hospitals, morgues, and related health services. Workers that share this classification include morgue attendants, child care attendants, and physical therapy aides.

What Are the Salary Ranges?

Although the salaries for most health care professionals vary by region and population, the average hourly wage of nurse assistants is about the same across the country. Midwestern states and less populated areas, where a large staff of nurse assistants may be needed to make up for a smaller staff of nurses and therapists, may pay a little more per hour.

Median weekly e arnings of full-time salaried nursing assistants were $292 in 1996. According to the Buck Survey conducted by the American health Care Association, nursing assistants in chain nursing homes had median hourly earnings of about $6.00 in 1996. The middle 50 percent earned betwen $5.95 and $7.50 per hour.

What Is the Job Outlook?

There will continue to be many job opportunities for nurse assistants. Because of the physical and emotional demands of the job, and because of the lack of advancement opportunities, there is a high turnover rate of employees. Also, health care is constantly changing; more opportunities open for nurse assistants as different kinds of health care facilities are developed. Business-based health organizations are limiting the services of health care professionals and looking for cheaper ways to provide care. This may provide opportunities for those looking for work as nurse assistants.

Government and private agencies are also developing more programs to assist dependent people. And as the number of people seventy years of age and older continues to rise, new and larger nursing care facilities will be needed.

Nurse-Midwife

SUMMARY

DEFINITION
A nurse-midwife is a registered nurse who assists in family planning, pregnancy, and childbirth. Nurse-midwives also provide routine health care for women.

ALTERNATIVE JOB TITLES
Certified Nurse-Midwife
Neonatal nurse

SALARY RANGE
$22,000 to $28,000 to $35,000+

EDUCATIONAL REQUIREMENTS
Two- to four-year registered nursing program; nine-month to two-year certified nurse-midwife program

CERTIFICATION OR LICENSING
Mandatory

EMPLOYMENT OUTLOOK
Faster than the average

HIGH SCHOOL SUBJECTS
Biology
Chemistry
English (writing/literature)
Philosophy
Psychology

PERSONAL INTERESTS
Helping people: emotionally
Helping people: physical health/medicine

The young woman found out last month that she was pregnant. It would be her second child. When she was pregnant the first time, three years ago, she was seeing an obstetrician for her prenatal care. She also had the obstetrician deliver her baby.

But she wanted to do things differently this time. Last time, she felt that she didn't receive the emotional support she needed from her doctor. And with all the pain killing drugs she was given during delivery, she almost felt as if she weren't in the room when her baby was born.

So this time she decided she was going to have a nurse-midwife give her prenatal care and deliver her baby. It would be a natural pregnancy and a natural childbirth. And now, after meeting with Deborah Woolley, her nurse-midwife, she knew she had made the right decision.

WHAT DOES A NURSE-MIDWIFE DO?

Midwifery, the act of assisting at childbirth, has been practiced around the world for thousands of years. But in the United States, pregnancy and childbirth are often considered technical medical procedures best left in the hands of physicians known as obstetricians and gynecologists. Midwifery has traditionally been frowned upon by both the medical community and the public.

WHAT DOES A NURSE-MIDWIFE DO?, CONTINUED

Since the 1960s, however, this attitude has been changing as more women insist on "natural" methods of giving birth. Nurse-midwives, officially known as certified nurse-midwives, have generally become accepted as respected members of health care teams involved with family planning, pregnancy, and childbirth. A number of studies have even indicated that babies delivered by nurse-midwives are less likely to experience low birth weights and other health complications than babies delivered by physicians.

Most nurse-midwives work at hospitals or at family planning clinics or birthing centers affiliated with hospitals. Some nurse-midwives operate independent practices providing home birth services.

Lingo to Learn

Catching babies: *An informal term used to describe the act of assisting in the delivery of an infant.*

Cesarean section: *A surgical procedure to deliver a baby through an incision in the abdomen. The procedure is named after Julius Caesar, who was supposedly born in this way.*

Episiotomy: *An incision made between the vagina and anus to provide more clearance for birth.*

Gynecologist: *A physician who specializes in the diseases and routine health care of the reproductive systems of women.*

Natural childbirth: *A term used to emphasize pregnancy, labor, and childbirth as natural processes. In natural childbirth, pain-reducing and labor-inducing drugs either are not used or are used conservatively.*

Obstetrician: *A physician who specializes in childbirth and in prenatal and postpartum care.*

Pap smear: *A procedure in which cells are collected from the cervix; the cells are then examined under a microscope for signs of cancer.*

Postpartum: *After childbirth.*

Prenatal: *Before childbirth.*

Nurse-midwives examine pregnant women and monitor the growth and development of fetuses. Typically, a nurse-midwife is responsible for all phases of a normal pregnancy, including prenatal care, assisting during labor, delivering the baby, and providing follow-up care. A nurse-midwife always works in consultation with a physician, who can be called upon should complications arise during pregnancy or childbirth. Nurse-midwives can provide emergency assistance to their patients while physicians are called. In most states, nurse-midwives are authorized to prescribe and administer medications. Many nurse-midwives provide the full spectrum of women's health care, including gynecological exams.

An important part of a nurse-midwife's work is concerned with the education of patients. Nurse-midwives teach their patients about proper nutrition and fitness for healthy pregnancies, and about different techniques for labor and delivery. Nurse-midwives also council their patients in the postpartum period—that is, after birth—about breast-feeding, parenting, and other areas concerning the health of mother and child. Nurse-midwives provide counseling on several other issues, including sexually transmitted diseases, spousal and child abuse, and social support networks. In some cases, counseling extends to patients' family members.

Not all midwives are certified nurse-midwives. Most states recognize other categories of midwives, including certified (or licensed) midwives and lay (or empirical) midwives.

//As a midwife, you have an impact not only on the birth experience, but also on all of a patient's life."

Certified midwives are not required to be nurses in order to practice as midwives. They typically assist in home births or at birthing centers, and are trained through a combination of formal education, apprenticeship, and self-education. Certified midwives are legally recognized in twenty-nine states, which offer licensing, certification, or registration programs. Certified midwives perform most of the services of nurse-midwives, and they generally have professional relationships with physicians, hospitals, and laboratories to provide support and emergency services.

Lay midwives usually obtain their training by apprenticing with established midwives, although some may acquire formal education as well. Lay midwives are midwives who are not certified or licensed, either because they lack the necessary experience and education or because they pursue nontraditional childbirth techniques. Many lay midwives practice only as part of religious communities or specific ethnic groups. Lay midwives typically assist only in home birth situations. Some states have made it illegal for lay midwives to charge for their services. The rest of this article will concern itself only with certified nurse-midwives.

WHAT IS IT LIKE TO BE A NURSE-MIDWIFE?

Deborah Woolley has been a registered nurse since 1975, and has been practicing as a nurse-midwife since 1983. She currently practices at the University of Illinois Hospital, where she also serves as the director of the university's Nurse-Midwifery Education Program. For Deborah, midwifery offered her the opportunity to have a positive impact on women's health care and childbirth experiences. "I started out as a nurse assigned to the labor and delivery unit. But I became frustrated with the type of care the women were getting," Deborah says. "You'll find that a lot among midwives. Most of the midwives I talk to can point to an event that was the straw that broke the camel's back, as it were, when they realized that they wanted to have more influence over the experience the woman is having. Midwifery's focus is on improving conditions for women and their families. In a way, midwifery is a radical departure from the old way of looking at pregnancy."

Deborah typically arrives at the hospital at 7:00 AM and spends the first hour or more seeing patients in postpartum—that is, women who have given birth the day or night before. At about 8:30, Deborah goes down to the clinic to begin seeing other patients. "I work a combination of full days and half days during the week. On a half day, I'll see patients for four hours and work on paperwork for one hour. On a full day, I'll see patients for eight hours and work on paperwork for two hours," Deborah says. "But that doesn't mean I always leave exactly at five o'clock. At the clinic, we see everyone who shows up."

After Deborah meets a new patient, she'll spend an hour or so taking the patient's medical history, examining her, and getting her scheduled into the prenatal care system. "I also ask about a patient's life. I spend time with the patient and try to get to know her and what's going on in her life. It makes a big difference in the care she's provided. I think one of the things that makes midwives so effective is that they really get to know their patients." Deborah points to one patient to highlight this. "One of my patients was a woman who was having her third child. This woman had always been good about keeping her appointments. Then she stopped coming in. I knew something had to be wrong. So I called people at different agencies, and they helped me track her down. It

Breast-feeding—benefits and bothers

Midwifery supports the practice of breast-feeding over bottle-feeding. Human milk contains antibodies that protect infants from infections, and breas-tfeeding strengthens the psychological bond between mother and child.

However, problems sometimes develop with breast-feeding. A breast may become engorged with milk, preventing the infant from sucking properly. In addition, nipples can become sore and cracked, and infections and abscesses can develop in the breasts.

Lactation consultants are health care professionals who help prevent and solve breast-feeding problems. They work in hospitals, public health centers, and private practices. The International Board of Lactation Consultant Examiners certifies lactation consultants.

Among the people certified as lactation consultants are many nurse-midwives, dieticians, physicians, and social workers.

Information about becoming a lactation consultant can be obtained from the International Lactation Consultant Association, 200 North Michigan Avenue, Suite 300, Chicago, IL 60601; Tel: 312-541-1710.

turned out that she had moved, and she wasn't doing well. We were able to get her back into the system and make sure she had a healthy baby."

Educating her patients is another part of the care Deborah provides. In fact, Deborah believes that education is one of a midwife's most important responsibilities. "I spend a lot of time teaching things like nutrition, the process of fetal development, and basic parenting skills. I'll refer patients to Lamaze classes. I'll also screen patients for family problems, such as violence in the home, and teach them how to get out of abusive situations," Deborah says. "In other words, I'll teach a patient anything she needs to know if she's pregnant. I try to empower women to take charge of their own health care and their own lives."

Apart from seeing patients, Deborah is also responsible for maintaining patients' records. "I have to review lab results and ultrasounds, and fill out birth certificates—things like that. I also have to make sure I have correct addresses on my patients," Deborah says. "There's a lot of writing involved, too. I have to document everything that I do with patients, including what I've done and how and why I've done it."

HAVE I GOT WHAT IT TAKES TO BE A NURSE-MIDWIFE?

"Speaking as both a midwife and someone who teaches midwives, I think there's one area that seems most difficult for some nurses who get into this profession," Deborah says. "That's making the leap from just being a physician's 'assistant' to having the autonomy of a midwife. As a midwife, you take on more responsibilities for the patient, and that means you have to be prepared to accept the consequences of the decisions you make. There is no more saying, 'I was only following orders,' if something goes wrong. Some nurses find that very stressful. But it's also part of what attracts a lot of us to this field. We really have a lot more direct influence on the quality and nature of our patients' care."

Midwifery is still not accepted by some physicians and other health care providers. "We don't get the slack that docs do," Deborah says. "A lot of people take a doctor's word as law. But a good midwife needs to know her business. She has to have a lot of infor-

To be a successful nurse-midwife, you should:

Enjoy working with people

Be independent and able to accept responsibility for your actions and decisions

Have strong observation, listening, and communication skills

Be confident and composed

mation at the top of her head—things like statistics, data, and procedures—and she needs to know exactly where that information comes from. This is because people still challenge a midwife's knowledge. And while a lot of obstetricians and gynecologists accept us, there are still many who don't. So you must be confident and poised when working with doctors."

Midwives share both in the joys of childbirth and in the tragedies. "The birth of children is supposed to be fun," Deborah says, "but the reality is that people also die. And in childbirth, when it goes bad, it goes really bad. I've had to hold babies while they die, and I've had to comfort mothers whose babies have died. This is especially difficult for midwives because they become so involved in their patients' lives. So anyone considering midwifery needs to be aware of this part of it, too. But again, most of us become midwives because of the real impact we can have on our patients and their childbirth experiences. It's a great job if you love it. And there really are many more ups than downs."

Giving her patients a sense of empowerment is one of the most important and most satisfying parts of Deborah's career. "Of course I love 'catching' [delivering] babies," Deborah says. "There's nothing as much fun as that. But over the course of my career I've gained more perspective, and I see now that that's not really where a midwife can make the most difference. The biggest part of what I do is to help women learn the stuff they need to make their own lives better. I've learned to ask a woman what she needs, and then to help her get it. The best is when I'm assisting a woman who's giving birth, and she looks up into my eyes and says, 'I did it.'"

FYI
Midwifery: Past and Present

The practice of midwifery is many thousands of years old. In most cultures around the world, births are usually attended to by midwives rather than physicians. The United States is one of the few countries where births are usually physician-delivered in hospital settings.

Hospitals began to replace homes as the places of birth early in the twentieth century. At the same time, the use of drugs to reduce pain and induce labor became commonplace. In addition, cesarean sections, in which the uterus is cut open for childbirth, increased in frequency.

Though this approach to childbirth undoubtedly decreased infant mortality in the United States, many people began to criticize it during the 1960s. The main criticism was that modern medicine was robbing women of the feelings and sensations associated with childbirth. The natural childbirth movement increased the popularity of midwifery.

Today, midwifery, as practiced by professional nurses who work in consultation with physicians, is generally accepted by the medical establishment.

Trying to empower patients can be very difficult. "There is a lot of frustration," Deborah acknowledges. "You're dealing with a lot of political and socioeconomic realities, like poverty, violence, and neglect, and this can become overwhelming at times. There's so much that needs to be done, and it's frustrating to recognize that you can't do it all. And these are aspects that cut across all levels of society. It's not just something that you face in a city hospital. It's in the suburbs and in rural areas, too." For Deborah and many midwives, however, this challenge is part of what brought them to this career. "As a midwife," Deborah says, "you have an impact not only on the birth experience, but also on all of a patient's life."

How Do I Become a Nurse-Midwife?

EDUCATION

High School

To prepare for a career in midwifery, high school students should focus on science courses. "I'd advise a high school student to take heavy science," Deborah says. "Those science courses may seem inapplicable at the time, but as you move into nursing you'll see how useful they actually are."

A prospective midwife needs to gain a broad range of education and experience. "A midwife is just as people-focused as she is science-focused," Deborah says. "So take courses in English, language, philosophy, psychology, and sociology. Language and communication skills are especially necessary because you'll be responsible for maintaining detailed reports on what you do with patients, and you'll be communicating information with patients, doctors, nurses, and insurance companies."

Deborah advises students to gain as much work experience as possible. "They should volunteer at hospitals, especially at facilities where they can work with adolescents. They can also become involved in peer-to-peer counseling." These experiences can make a difference in gaining admission into a midwifery program.

Postsecondary Training

All nurse-midwives begin their careers as registered nurses. In order to become a registered nurse, you must first graduate from either a four-year bachelor's degree program in nursing or a two-year associate's degree program in nursing. After receiving a degree, you will need to apply for admission into an accredited certificate program in nurse-midwifery or an accredited master's degree program in nurse-midwifery.

If you have earned an associate's degree in nursing, you are eligible for acceptance into a certificate program in nurse-midwifery. A certificate program requires nine to twelve months of study. In order to be accepted into a master's degree program in nurse-midwifery, you will need a bachelor's degree in nursing. A master's degree program requires sixteen to twenty-four months of study. Some master's degree programs also require one year of clinical experience in order to earn a degree as a nurse-midwife. In these programs, you will be trained to provide primary care services, gynecological care, preconception and prenatal care, labor delivery and management, and postpartum and infant care.

As you train to become a nurse-midwife you will also learn how to perform physical examinations, Pap smears, and episiotomies, as well as repair incisions from cesarean sections; administer anesthesia; and prescribe medications. You will also be trained to provide counseling on such subjects as nutrition, breastfeeding, and infant care, as well as emotional support.

CERTIFICATION OR LICENSING

After graduating from a nurse-midwifery program, you will be required to take a national examination administered by the American College of Nurse-Midwives (ACNM). When you pass this examination you will be licensed to practice nurse-midwifery in all fifty states. Each state, however, has its own laws and regulations governing the activities and responsibilities of nurse-midwives.

WHO WILL HIRE ME?

Deborah earned a bachelor's degree in nursing and then began her career as a nurse at a labor and delivery unit in a Texas hospital. While working, she attended graduate school and received a master's degree in maternal child nursing. She then came to Chicago, where she began training as a nurse-midwife. "After earning my nurse-midwifery degree," Deborah says, "I heard there were openings at Cook County Hospital here in Chicago. So I applied for a job there. What I liked about Cook County was that they continued to train me while I was working. They gave me assertiveness training and training in urban health issues."

Hospitals are the primary source of employment for nurse-midwives. Approximately 85 percent of the more than 6,000 nurse-midwives in the United States work in hospitals. Most of the remaining nurse-midwives work in family planning clinics (including Planned Parenthood centers) and other health care clinics and agencies. Some nurse-midwives operate their own clinics and birthing centers, while others work independently and specialize in home birth deliveries.

WHERE CAN I GO FROM HERE?

With experience, a nurse-midwife can advance into a supervisory role or into an administrative capacity at a hospital, family planning clinic, birthing center, or other facility. Many nurse-midwives, like Deborah, choose to continue their education and complete Ph.D. programs. With a doctorate, a nurse-midwife can do research or teaching. "I spent four-and-a-half years at Cook County while I was working on my Ph.D.," Deborah says. "Then I was recruited to Colorado to head up the midwifery unit at a hospital there. After six years as a director in Colorado, I learned that the director's position here at UIC was open, and I jumped at the chance to come back to Chicago."

Related Jobs

Community health nurses

Directors of nursing services

Directors of schools of nursing

Nurse anesthetists

Nurse practitioners

Office nurses

Private and general duty nurses

School nurses

WHAT ARE SOME RELATED JOBS?

The U.S. Department of Labor classifies nurse-midwives with others in nursing occupations. Among these workers are nurse anesthetists, private and general duty nurses, nurse practitioners, and school nurses. The U.S. Department of Labor also classifies nurse-midwives with other registered nurses. Among these workers are office nurses, directors of nursing services, directors of schools of nursing, and community health nurses.

WHAT ARE THE SALARY RANGES?

The median salary for an experienced nurse-midwife was about $70,100 per year in 1996, accoring to a Hay Group survey of HMOs, group practices, and hospital-based clinics. The middle 50 percent earned between $59,300 and $75,700. Starting salaries for beginning nurse-midwives range from $22,000 to $28,000 per year, depending on the place of employment; those working for large hospitals tend to earn more than those working for small hospitals, clinics, and birthing centers. Salaries also vary according to the region of the country; according to urban, suburban, or rural setting; and according to whether the employing facility is private or public.

WHAT ARE THE SALARY RANGES?, CONTINUED

Nurse-midwives generally enjoy a good benefits package, although these too can vary widely. Most nurse-midwives work a forty-hour week. The hours are sometimes irregular, involving working at night and on weekends. This is partly due to the fact that the timing of natural childbirth cannot be controlled.

WHAT IS THE JOB OUTLOOK?

The number of nurse-midwifery jobs is expected to grow faster than the average for all occupations through 2006, as nurse-midwives gain a reputation as an integral part of the health care community. Currently, there are more positions than there are nurse-midwives to fill them. This situation is expected to continue for the near future.

There are two factors driving the demand for nurse-midwives. The first factor is the growth of interest in natural childbearing techniques among women. The number of midwife-assisted births has risen dramatically since the 1970s. Some women have been attracted to midwifery because of studies that indicate natural childbirth is more healthful for mother and child than doctor-assisted childbirth. Other women have been attracted to midwifery because it emphasizes the participation of the entire family in prenatal care and labor.

The second factor in the growing demand for nurse-midwives is economic in nature. As society moves toward managed-care programs and the health care community emphasizes cost-effectiveness, midwifery should increase in popularity. This is because the care provided by nurse-midwives costs substantially less than the care provided by obstetricians and gynecologists. If the cost advantage of midwifery continues, more insurers and health maintenance organizations will probably direct patients to nurse-midwives for care.

Nurse Practitioner

SUMMARY

DEFINITION
Nurse practitioners *are registered nurses (RNs) who have advanced education in diagnosis and treatment that enables them to carry out many health care responsibilities formerly handled by physicians.*

ALTERNATIVE JOB TITLES
Family nurse practitioner
Gerontological nurse practitioner
Occupational health nurse practitioner
Pediatric nurse practitioner
Psychiatric nurse practitioner
School nurse practitioner

SALARY RANGE
$40,000 to $47,432 to $70,000+

EDUCATIONAL REQUIREMENTS
Master's degree

CERTIFICATION OR LICENSING
Licensing as an RN is mandatory; additional certification for nurse practitioners is recommended.

EMPLOYMENT OUTLOOK
Faster than the average

HIGH SCHOOL SUBJECTS
Biology
Chemistry
English (writing/literature)
Mathematics

PERSONAL INTERESTS
Helping people: emotionally
Helping people: physical health/medicine

In working with college students, Harvey Bennett says it is essential to establish rapport. "You need to be a good listener and make it clear that confidentiality will be respected," he explains.

Harvey, the head nurse practitioner at Vanderbilt University's Student Health Service, spends much of his workday seeing students with a variety of health complaints. An average of 150 students visit the Health Service each day, with problems ranging from colds and sore throats to alcohol-related problems or eating disorders.

Careful assessment of each case is important. Most of the time, it turns out that one of the Center's six nurse practitioners can handle the problem without calling in a staff physician.

WHAT DOES A NURSE PRACTITIONER DO?

Nurse practitioners provide health care in a wide range of settings, generally focusing on primary care, health maintenance, and prevention of illness. They carry out many of the medical responsibilities traditionally handled by physi-

WHAT DOES A NURSE PRACTITIONER DO?, CONTINUED

cians. They do physical exams, take detailed medical histories, order lab tests and X rays, and recommend treatment plans.

The nurse practitioner role developed in the 1960s in response to the shortage of physicians and the need for alternative health care providers, especially in remote rural areas. Harvey Bennett was attracted to the profession during its early years because he valued its goal—to keep people out of the hospital by providing good primary and preventive care.

As a result of their advanced training, nurse practitioners are qualified to work more autonomously than staff nurses. In 1986, a study carried out by the U.S. Congress Office of Technology Assessment found that "within their areas of competence, nurse practitioners provide care whose quality is equivalent to that of care provided by physicians." In preventive care and communication with patients, nurse practitioners were found to surpass doctors. By 1992, there were approximately thirty thousand nurse practitioners in the United States, and the number is continuing to increase rapidly.

A nurse practitioner's exact responsibilities depend on the setting in which she or he works and the field of specialization chosen. A nurse practitioner may work in close collaboration with a physician at a hospital, health center, or private practice office or, as in the case of a rural health care provider, may have only weekly telephone contact with a physician. Nurse practitioners may not function entirely independently of a physician, although the degree of consultation required varies from state to state. As Harvey points out, it is important for nurse practitioners to develop the judgment to recognize when an illness or injury is beyond their level of competence.

Most nurse practitioners have a field of specialization. The commonest specialty (and the broadest in its scope) is *family nurse practitioner (FNP)*. Family nurse practitioners, who

Lingo to Learn

Acute: *Describes a disease or symptom that begins suddenly and does not last long.*

Advanced practice nurses: *Nurses with advanced education that enables them to take on many responsibilities formerly carried out by physicians; nurse practitioners, clinical nurse specialists, certified nurse midwives, and certified registered nurse anesthetists are classed as advanced practice nurses.*

Chronic: *Describes a disease or condition that develops gradually and often remains for the rest of the person's life, such as glaucoma.*

Clinical: *Pertaining to direct, hands-on medical care; from the Greek word for "bed."*

Licensed practical nurse (LPN): *An individual trained in basic nursing who usually works under the supervision of a registered nurse.*

Pap smear: *A test that examines cells (taken during a pelvic exam) to detect cancers of the cervix.*

Protocol: *A written plan (prepared in advance) that details the procedures to be followed in providing care for a particular medical condition.*

Wellness: *A dynamic state of health in which a person moves toward higher levels of functioning—a term often used by NPs.*

are often based in community health clinics, provide primary care to people of all ages—assessing, diagnosing, and treating common illnesses and injuries. Their interactions with patients have a strong emphasis on teaching and counseling for health maintenance. Nurse practitioners recognize the importance of the social and emotional aspects of health care, in addition to the more obvious physical factors.

//Within their areas of competence, nurse practitioners provide care whose quality is equivalent to that of care provided by physicians."

Nurse practitioners in other specialties perform similar tasks, though working with different age groups or with people in school, workplace, or institutional settings. *Pediatric nurse practitioners (PNPs)* provide primary health care for children (infants through adolescents). Developmental assessment is an important part of the pediatric nurse practitioner's responsibilities: Is this child within the norms of physical and social growth for his or her age group? *Gerontological nurse practitioners (GNPs)* work with older adults. They are often based in nursing homes.

School nurse practitioners work in school settings and provide primary health care for students in elementary, secondary, or higher education settings. *Occupational health nurse practitioners* focus on employment-related health problems and injuries. They work closely with occupational health physicians, toxicologists, safety specialists, and other occupational health professionals to identify potential dangers and to prevent work-related illness or injury. *Psychiatric nurse practitioners* work with people who have mental or emotional problems.

Women's health care nurse practitioners provide primary care for women from adolescence through old age. In addition to handling overall primary care, they do Pap smears and breast exams, provide information on family planning and birth control, monitor normal pregnancies, and offer treatment and counseling for gynecological problems and sexually transmitted diseases. Some nurse practitioners are also certified in midwifery.

In most states, nurse practitioners are allowed to write certain prescriptions, but a physician's signature is often required to validate it.

WHAT IS IT LIKE TO BE A NURSE PRACTITIONER?

Harvey Bennett has been a nurse practitioner in Vanderbilt's Student Health Service since 1984. He is certified as a family nurse practitioner. Though he is qualified to provide primary care to persons of all ages, in his present position his practice is confined to the Vanderbilt student population—undergraduates who are generally eighteen to twenty-two and graduate and professional students who may be in their twenties, thirties, and forties.

After completing the nurse practitioner program at Vanderbilt, Harvey spent six years working as a family nurse practitioner based in rural health clinics in Alabama and Georgia. Each clinic was staffed by a nurse practitioner; there was a physician "somewhere in the county." During his Georgia years, the nearest hospital was thirty-five miles away. The shortage of doctors and hospitals meant that the nurse practitioners formed long-term relationships with the people they served and had the satisfaction of knowing that they were making a difference in people's lives. It also meant that they were likely to have people knocking on the door in the middle of the night with a medical emergency. In both Alabama and Georgia, Harvey found a high level of acceptance from patients, but in Alabama there was considerable hostility to nurse practitioners from the medical establishment. During the Reagan administration, clinic funding was cut back, so Harvey returned to Nashville.

At Student Health, Harvey spends most of his time seeing students who have come in with health problems. He takes a history from each patient, does a physical, and orders lab tests (if indicated). Treatment is based on a protocol developed by the nurse practitioners and doctors; as long as the complaint can be handled within the protocol, the nurse practitioner works without consulting the doctor.

In assessing each case, it is essential to find out whether the reported symptoms may actually reflect a more serious underlying problem. For example, in many cases, students suffering from depression come to the Center complaining of headaches, stomach pains, or fatigue.

Teaching and counseling are important parts of the job. College students are at a formative age, and Harvey tries to make a positive impact on their daily health habits. Health topics he discusses with them include alcohol and tobacco use, diet, seat-belt use, and the need to wear bicycle safety helmets. Students often need assistance in making the connection between the symptoms they are experiencing and their behavior (such as smoking or excessive consumption of alcohol). In addition to seeing patients, Harvey, as head nurse practitioner, is also responsible for scheduling and quality control.

Another area of specialization is gerontological nursing care. Kay Grott spent about seven years as a gerontological nurse practitioner in several Tennessee nursing homes. She first encountered this specialty in a junior-year seminar during her undergraduate nursing program at East Tennessee State University. At that time, the lack of appropriate health care for older adults had become a focus of public concern, and Kay decided that she wanted to contribute to solving the problem.

FYI

The nurse practitioner role developed in the 1960s in response to the shortage of physicians and the need for alternative health care providers.

At first, she planned to become a clinical nurse specialist with a concentration in gerontological care, but one of her instructors urged her to become a nurse practitioner instead; he pointed out that nurse practitioners were assuming an increasingly important role in the health care industry. Receiving her MS from the Medical College of Virginia, Kay found the nurse practitioner role to be a "good fit."

As a nurse practitioner at a nursing home, Kay was the person responsible for coordinating her patients' total care. She was the liaison between the patient's family, the physician, and the other health care providers. Good communication skills are essential, as well as being comfortable working with older people; that part was easy for Kay, who grew up in an extended multigenerational family. Her work included taking detailed medical histories of each patient, performing physical exams, ordering lab tests and X rays, and monitoring chronic illnesses. It is also important to monitor the patient's progress under the treatment plan drawn up by the health care team. Some typical medical problems are Alzheimer's disease, Parkinson's disease, cardiac conditions, and COPD (Chronic Obstructive Pulmonary Diseases).

Working with people approaching the end of life, Kay often had to deal with issues of death and dying. Sometimes that meant helping to make people's last months as peaceful and comfortable as possible instead of pursuing an aggressive treatment plan.

A nurse practitioner employed at a nursing home is not always involved in direct patient care. At one point, Kay worked as director of nursing. In that position, she succeeded in raising the nursing home's standards of care to meet new federal standards introduced in the late 1980s.

HAVE I GOT WHAT IT TAKES TO BE A NURSE PRACTITIONER?

A nurse practitioner needs to enjoy working with people and to be strongly committed to making a positive difference in people's lives. Nurse practitioners must develop excellent communication skills. Being a good listener is essential, as is the ability to encourage people to answer questions about personal matters that they may find difficult to talk about. Anyone going into the health care field needs to have patience and flexibility and the ability to remain calm in an emergency.

Since nurse practitioners work more independently than nurses traditionally do, it is important for them to develop the capacity to take active responsibility in health care situations. At the same time, they must have the judgment to identify those situations that are beyond their competence and to call in a physician or other specialist.

Because the nurse practitioner role is strongly focused on health maintenance and prevention, a person considering becoming a nurse practitioner should find teaching and counseling at least as satisfying as dramatic medical interventions.

A nurse practitioner has to be prepared for the possibility of friction with professional colleagues. The nurse-practitioner profession is still new, and some physicians are uncomfortable with it; some display hostility to the idea of nurses functioning in autonomous roles. The nurse practitioner seems to be perceived as a threat by some physicians. Relations with staff nurses can also be a problem for nurse practitioners at times, because some staff nurses resent taking orders from anyone except a doctor. Some patients who have never encountered a nurse practitioner before may be concerned about "just seeing the nurse instead of the doctor." All these situations need to be handled in a mature and professional way.

The problems involved in dealing with insurance companies are also a major source of stress for many nurse practitioners. Although the nurse practitioner is widely recognized as a cost-effective provider of health care, insurance regulations make it difficult for them to receive direct reimbursement.

*To be a **successful** nurse **practitioner**, you should:*

Be strongly committed to making a positive difference in people's lives

Have patience and the ability to remain calm in an emergency

Find teaching and counseling as satisfying as dramatic medical interventions

Be able to identify those medical situations where it is necessary to call in a physician

HOW DO I BECOME A NURSE PRACTITIONER?

EDUCATION

High School

Future nurse practitioners should take a well-balanced college preparatory course in high school, with a good foundation in the sciences. Obviously, biology, chemistry, and physics are important courses. If your high school offers anatomy and physiology as a follow-up to the basic biology course, that would be a good elective. You also need to take courses in the humanities and social sciences. Classes that improve communication skills are especially helpful for anyone going into a people-oriented field like nursing.

The high school years are also a good time to start getting some hands-on experience in health care. Try doing volunteer work at a local hospital, community health center, or nursing home. There are probably nurse practitioners in your community who would be glad to discuss their work with you and let you follow them around for a few days to observe.

Postsecondary Training

You need to be a registered nurse (RN) before you may become a nurse practitioner. There are three ways to become an RN: an associate's degree program at a junior or community college, a diploma program at a hospital school of nursing, or a bachelor's-degree program at a college or university. All programs combine classroom study and clinical experience in hospitals and other health care settings.

A bachelor's degree is generally necessary for anyone who wants to go on for the additional training (usually a master's degree) required to become a nurse practitioner. A student who begins nursing study in an associate's degree or diploma program may transfer into a bachelor's degree program later. Students with an undergraduate major other than nursing may also enter nursing degree programs, although they may need to fulfill some additional prerequisites. (Harvey Bennett has an undergraduate degree in engineering. After serving in the Navy in the Vietnam War, he decided that he wanted to find a different profession.)

In nursing school, students study the theory and practice of nursing, taking such courses as human anatomy and physiology, psychology, microbiology, nutrition, and statistics. Students in bachelor's degree programs also study English, humanities, and social sciences. After finishing their educational program, students must pass a national examination in order to be licensed to practice nursing in their state and to use the initials "RN" after their name.

HOW DO I BECOME A . . . ?, CONTINUED

A master's degree is usually required to become a nurse practitioner. Programs last one to two years and provide advanced study in diagnostic skills, health assessment, pharmacology, clinical management, and research skills. Classroom work is combined with "hands-on" clinical practice. Usually the student begins with generalist work and later focuses on preparation for a specific nurse practitioner specialty. Admission to good nurse practitioner programs is very competitive.

CERTIFICATION OR LICENSING

Every state requires RNs to pass the National Council Licensing Examination before they are allowed to practice in that state. Some states require continuing education for license renewal.

National certification exams for nurse practitioners are available and strongly recommended by professional organizations, although not every state requires nurse practitioners to have national certification.

WHO WILL HIRE ME?

Nurse practitioners are employed in hospitals, clinics, physicians' offices, community health centers, rural health clinics, nursing homes, mental health centers, educational institutions, student health centers, nursing schools, home health agencies, hospices, prisons, industrial organizations, the U.S. military, and other health care settings. In the states that allow nurse practitioners to practice independently, self-employment is an option.

The particular specialty you pursue is obviously a major factor in determining your employment setting. Another important factor is the degree of autonomy you desire. Nurse practitioners in remote rural areas have the most autonomy, but they must be willing to spend a lot of time on the road visiting patients who are unable to get to the clinic, to be on call at all hours, and to make do with less than optimal facilities and equipment.

The placement office of your nursing school is a good place to begin the employment search. Contacts you have made in clinical settings during your nurse practitioner program are also useful sources of information on job opportunities. Nursing registries, nurse employment services, and your state employment office have information about available jobs. Nursing journals and newspapers list openings. If you are interested in working for the federal government, contact the Office of Personnel Management for your region.

Applying directly to hospitals, nursing homes, and other health care agencies is also an option for nurse practitioners.

WHERE CAN I GO FROM HERE?

Nurse practitioners have many avenues for advancement. After gaining experience, they may move into positions that offer more responsibility and higher salaries. Some choose to move into administrative or supervisory positions in health care organizations or nursing schools. They may become faculty members at nursing schools or directors of nursing at a hospital, clinic, or other health agency.

Some advance by doing additional academic and clinical study that gives them certification in specialized fields. Those with an interest in research, teaching, consulting, or policy-making in the nursing field would do well to consider earning a Ph.D. in nursing. In the early 1990s, there were thirty-three doctoral degree programs in nursing in the United States, and that number seems likely to increase.

WHAT ARE SOME RELATED JOBS?

The U.S. Department of Labor classifies nurse practitioners and other registered nurses with people in the "Health Assessment and Treating Occupations," a sub-category of the much broader "Professional Speciality Occupations" field. Also under the "Health Assessment and Treating Occupations" heading are dietitians and nutritionists, pharmacists, occupational therapists, recreational therapists, respiratory therapists, physicians' assistants, audiologists, and speech-language pathologists.

Related Jobs

Community health nurses
Directors of nursing services
Directors of schools of nursing
Nurse anesthetists
Nurse-midwives
Office nurses
Private and general duty nurses
School nurses

WHAT ARE THE SALARY RANGES?

In 1996, nurse practitioners' salaries ranged from the low $40,000s to over $70,000, with the median estimated to be $47,432, according to a recent University of Texas Medical Branch survey. Geographical location and experi-

WHAT ARE THE SALARY RANGES?, CONTINUED

ence are factors in salary levels. Nurse practitioners should expect to frequently work long and inconvenient hours, especially if they are in rural practice.

WHAT IS THE JOB OUTLOOK?

The job outlook for nurse practitioners is excellent, since the nurse practitioner is being increasingly recognized as a provider of the high-quality yet cost-effective medical care that the nation's health care system needs. More and more, people are recognizing the importance of preventive health care, which, of course, is one of the nurse practitioner's greatest strengths. All nurse practitioner specialties are expected to continue growing. There should be an especially strong demand for gerontological nurse practitioners, as the percentage of the U.S. population in the over-sixty-five age group increases. The Midwest and the South are expected to be the areas of greatest growth in demand for nurse practitioners.

Nurse practitioner organizations are working to promote legislation that will increase the degree of autonomy available to nurse practitioners and make it easier for them to receive insurance company reimbursement. This should make the profession an even more attractive route of advancement for RNs.

At the same time, it is important for those entering the profession to have realistic expectations. Some nurse practitioners report increasing frustration with recent cutbacks in the health care industry that make it difficult to persuade insurance companies to approve for reimbursement the treatment plans considered necessary by health care professionals. Problems with insurance companies and current restrictions on autonomy lead to burnout and disillusionment for some nurse practitioners, who emerged from their master's degree programs with idealistic goals for their profession.

Registered Nurse

SUMMARY

DEFINITION
Registered nurses (RNs) *administer medical care to sick or injured individuals and help people achieve health and prevent disease.*

ALTERNATIVE JOB TITLES
Staff nurses

SALARY RANGE
$20,000 to $40,000 to $55,000+

EDUCATIONAL REQUIREMENTS
Associate's degree through an accredited junior college; diploma from a nursing school; bachelor's degree

CERTIFICATION OR LICENSING
Mandatory

EMPLOYMENT OUTLOOK
Faster than the average

HIGH SCHOOL SUBJECTS
Biology
English (writing/literature)
Mathematics

PERSONAL INTERESTS
Helping people: emotionally
Helping people: physical health/medicine

It's three in the morning in the intensive care unit. Nurses on the night shift are making their rounds, listening to the instruments that monitor their patients, changing IV bags, or giving medicine. In the emergency room several cases come in all at once; even though they are seven hours into their shift, the trauma nurses immediately snap to in a flurry of activity. Their ability to react quickly and make decisions under pressure can make the difference between life or death.

Meanwhile, at a retirement community not far away, a live-in nurse assists her client to the bathroom, walking slowly to help her navigate the long hallway from her bedroom safely. Although it is eleven o'clock at night, the nurse shows no hint of irritation or fatigue. It is her job to help her patient in any way she can.

WHAT DOES A REGISTERED NURSE DO?

Just as the title "doctor" encompasses numerous specialties and branches of study, the title "registered nurse" is an umbrella term, covering many different aspects of nursing. Although nurses work in various health care facilities, they have three basic goals: to assist the ill, disabled, or elderly in the recovery or maintenance of life functions; to prevent illness and relapse of illness; and to

79

promote health in the community. Most nurses come into contact with patients more frequently than other members of the health care community. Doctors are busy with diagnosis and the creation of treatment plans, and often do not have time to carry out the plans themselves. Because of this, nurses often provide the human element in a patient's treatment. They observe a patient's symptoms and evaluate progress or lack of progress. Nurses are also responsible for educating their patients and families on how to cope with a long-term illness or disability.

The field of nursing is broken down by the setting in which a nurse works. A registered nurse typically works under the guidance of a physician, who will develop a care plan for a patient that the nurse helps to administer. But the specific work of each nurse can take many forms. *General duty nurses* offer bedside nursing care and observe the progress of the patients. They may also supervise licensed practical nurses and aides. *Surgical nurses* are part of a logistical team in the operating room that supports the surgeon. They sterilize instruments, prepare patients for surgery, and coordinate the transfer of patients to and from the operating room. A *maternity nurse* looks after newborn infants, assists in the delivery room, and educates new mothers and fathers on basic child care. A *head nurse* directs and coordinates the activities of the nursing staff. Other hospital staff nurses are trained to work in intensive care units, the emergency room, and in the pediatric ward.

Registered nurses work in varied settings. *Home health nurses* provide nursing care, prescribed by a physician, to patients at home. They assist a wide range of patients, such as those recovering from illnesses and accidents, and must be able to work independently. *Private duty nurses* may work in hospitals or in a patient's home. They are employed by the patient they are caring for or by the patient's family. Their duties are carried out in cooperation with the patient's physician.

Office nurses work in clinics or at the private practice of a physician. Their duties may combine nursing skills—taking blood pressure, assisting with

Lingo to Learn

Case manager: *A nurse or administrator who coordinates the medical care of a patient.*

Crash cart: *The cart that carries medicines, equipment, and machines that may be needed in an emergency situation in an intensive care unit or emergency room.*

Intubate: *To insert breathing apparatus into the throat of a patient who is unable to breathe satisfactorily.*

Nursing home: *A long-term care facility that provides the elderly and chronically ill with health care and assistance with daily activities, such as bathing, eating, and dressing.*

Skilled nursing facility: *A facility that provides round-the-clock medical care by registered nurses and other licensed health care professionals.*

Vital signs: *The pulse rate, breathing rate, and body temperature of a person.*

outpatient procedures, patient education—with administrative or office duties such as scheduling appointments, keeping files, and answering phones. Nurses in this field may work for a Health Maintenance Organization (HMO) or an insurance company.

Nursing home nurses direct the care of residents in long-term care facilities. The work is similar to that done in hospitals; however, a nursing home nurse cares for patients with conditions ranging from a hip fracture to Parkinson's disease. *Public health nurses,* or *community health nurses,* work with government and private agencies to educate the public about health care issues. Their work might include creating a community blood pressure testing site, speaking about nutrition and disease, and providing immunizations and disease screenings for members of their community. Many school children are screened by public health nurses for such conditions as poor vision and scoliosis.

Occupational health nurses, or *industrial nurses,* provide nursing care in a clinic at a work site. They provide emergency care, work on accident prevention programs, and offer health counseling.

WHAT IS IT LIKE TO BE A REGISTERED NURSE?

"A lot of people see nursing as bedpans and sponge baths, but that isn't the case anymore." Jen Macri works in an intensive care unit (ICU) on second shift at Christ Center and Medical Hospital in Oak Lawn. Her workday runs from about 3:00 to 11:00 PM, four days a week. Although she acknowledges that new nurses often get night and evening shifts, she points out that that isn't necessarily a bad thing. "I like second shift because it doesn't interrupt my sleep patterns. Some people like the rush of first shift—there's always a lot going on then. Some people really like nights, and wouldn't give them up for anything. Night staff are a special breed." Because most of the hospital administrative staff goes home at the end of the first shift, hospitals usually quiet down during second shift; fewer nurses are assigned to night and evening duty.

Jen's regular duties in the ICU include administering medicines that patients are supposed to receive. "Any kind of patient care—bathing, changing linens, monitoring support systems—that is also our responsibility. We do all the things nurses in other parts of the hospital do for their patients." What makes the ICU different is its uncertainty. Jen's patients are stable but monitored. "If a patient becomes unstable, we address the problem ourselves—we

can't just call for a doctor and wait for him to show up. We have to begin dealing with the situation ourselves."

Nurses often provide a human element to hospital stays. Because of the
life-threatening conditions of her patients, comfort and support for concerned
family members is a significant part of Jen's day. "Sometimes you'll end up
doing part of the doctor's job. The doctor might sit the family down and explain
a condition to them and they nod their heads, 'Yes, Doctor,' and have no idea
what he was talking about. You kind of have to interpret what the doctor meant
for people; you are more accessible to the patient and to the family than the
doctors usually are."

Jen also finds that ICU nurses are allowed a certain freedom that is not
usual on the other floors. "The doctors rely on us pretty heavily to keep track of
patient status," she notes, and with the added responsibility comes an added
amount of independence. Additionally, some ICU nurses may find that the
restrictions placed on other hospital nurses by insurance companies or administrative staff are lessened for them, because of the immediate and critical
nature of the care they provide.

//When you know you've done something caring to help someone else, you know you've done well."

Jen works with about ten other nurses per shift, and in her ICU there
are twenty-two beds, so the nurse-to-patient ratio is about one to two. In other
parts of the hospital, this ratio can be one to five or as high as one to twenty-
five, depending on the type of care that is required and on the shift that is being
scheduled. The general trend in hospitals is toward a higher nurse-to-patient
ratio, which makes nurses responsible for more patients at a time. Jen works
overtime if she is in the midst of a situation that has occurred on her shift. "You
don't just go home when the shift is over. If somebody goes unstable in the last
half hour of your shift, it is still your responsibility to handle it."

Nursing demands alertness, education, and a certain amount of mental and physical stamina. "Intensive care can be stressful physically, because
you are moving people who aren't able to move themselves. And it can be mentally tiring, too, because you see a lot of sickness and death. Not everybody
dying is eighty, either; I have seen twenty- and thirty-year olds in ICU."
Occasionally, nurses in Jen's unit will have a debriefing to help them cope with

a traumatic event or a death in their unit. "The people that you work with are so supportive—it's kind of the nature of the job. You really have to be there for each other."

Like other aspects of health care, nursing has become increasingly cost-conscious and somewhat political in recent years. Some nurses have a difficult time adjusting to the requirements of insurance companies and administrators, and resent the fact that they are allowed less contact with their patients than before. Because Jen is new to nursing, she was trained with the current health care issues in mind, and finds that she is not as critical about some requirements as some of her older co-workers.

HAVE I GOT WHAT IT TAKES TO BE A REGISTERED NURSE?

To be a successful nurse, says Jen Macri, you have to be adept at problem-solving. "You have to be pretty organized, especially now that [hospital administration] is laying more and more in your lap and you have less time to do everything." More than anything else, nurses must be genuinely concerned for the people with whom they are working. "Ultimately, you're there to do good for the people," Jen summarizes. "People who aren't into that don't last very long."

Bunny Sendelbach, a nurse of almost twenty years, agrees. Bunny currently works in a retirement community where she provides care to elderly residents. "A nurse should be someone who has an aptitude in science, psychology, and who knows how to get along with a huge team. Most of all, you have to be able to inspire confidence and make your patients feel secure and good about themselves. That's the key to good health." Bunny feels that nursing is really still a calling, though this can be in the increasingly technical and financial aspects of the work. "To be a good

To be a successful registered nurse, you should:

Have keen observational skills

Be able to work under pressure

Follow orders precisely

Be well organized

Be caring and sympathetic

Handle emergencies calmly

healer, you have to be able to put aside your own ego, and give patients the best environment you can so they can heal themselves. Nurses have to have heart, but they have to have brains as well."

The benefits of nursing are not limited to patients. Asked what made nursing worth the emotional stress and responsibility, Jen answered immediately. She appreciates the gratitude of patients and family; she also appreciates being able to contribute. "It's the people that get well and come back to say thank you, even if you only did a little smidge of something. You feel like you contributed by helping somebody. That's well worth everything else. When you know you've done something caring to help somebody else, you know you've done well." Patience, tact, and efficiency are qualities that make a good nurse. A strong sense of purpose and courage are qualities that will keep a good nurse in the career for years to come.

HOW DO I BECOME A REGISTERED NURSE?

EDUCATION

High School
While still in high school, take core science and math classes, including biology, chemistry, and physics. Other classes to take include psychology and sociology. Communication skills are vital to successful nurses, so English and speech courses will be useful.

It is possible to volunteer in many of the places nurses work, in order to decide if nursing is the career you want. Hospitals will take on high school volunteers as candy stripers or assistants, delivering mail and flowers, visiting with patients, and doing routine office work. While volunteerships at this level are not really concerned with patient treatment, they enable the prospective nurse to understand the way the hospital works and who is responsible for what duty.

While volunteering, you may be given more opportunity as a technician or as an aide to contribute to patient care. In many cases, according to Jen, if hospitals know you are seriously considering a career in nursing, they will give you better opportunities for hands-on involvement and experiences. "They'll say, come in here and help intubate Mr. So-and-So. One of the great things about being a volunteer is that it can be a direct line into a job at that hospital." Hospitals have a vested interest in training people to be nurses, especially if it means they will be able to hire somebody who is already familiar with the workings of their administration and setup.

Postsecondary Training
There are three training programs for registered nurses: associate's degree programs, diploma programs, and bachelor's degree programs. All three programs combine classroom education with actual nursing experience. Associate's degrees in nursing usually involve a two-year program at a junior or commu-

nity college that is affiliated with a hospital. Many Associate's Degree Nurses (ADN) seek further schooling in bachelor's programs after they have found employment, in order to take advantage of tuition reimbursement programs.

FYI

The first U.S. school of nursing was established in 1872 at the New England Hospital for Women and Children in Boston.

The diploma program is conducted through independent nursing schools and teaching hospitals. This program usually lasts three years, and is the type that Jen went through and heartily recommends. "There are big differences in the programs. I think the best ones are done from big teaching hospitals, where you have the opportunities to see things that you wouldn't see in community hospitals or in associate's degree programs. I saw things at Rush (Presbyterian-St. Luke's Hospital in Chicago) that I would never have seen in a suburban hospital, and will probably never see again."

A bachelor's degree (BSN) is recommended for nurses who must compete in an era of cutbacks and small staffs. Additionally, bachelor's degree programs are recommended for those who may want to go into administration or supervision. It is also required for jobs in public health agencies and for admission to graduate school.

CERTIFICATION OR LICENSING

Those who pass an accredited nursing program are known as nurse graduates, but must still pass the licensing exam to become a Registered Nurse. Licensing is required in all fifty states, and license renewal or continuing education credits are also required periodically. In some cases, licensing in one state will automatically grant licensing in reciprocal states.

You will need additional training if you wish to advance into specialized practices, administration, and teaching. This may include further clinical training within the hospital in an area such as pediatrics or gerontology, or entering a master's degree program.

WHO WILL HIRE ME?

Jen believes that belonging to an association makes you more marketable to employers because it increases your awareness of what is happening in the nursing community. "I joined an association to put it on my resume, but the magazines they sent me ended up being really helpful and interesting. They keep you up-to-date with new practices, and also advancements in the medical community and what that means to nursing. They have articles about medicine written for the lay person; they aren't written like medical trade journals. And managers love to see that stuff on applications—they know it keeps you aware and informed."

As with most jobs, persistence pays off, and special education can be a key element in winning specific jobs. "Right out of school I started knocking on doors. I wanted to work in the Surgical Heart Unit (SHU). I had extra cardiac training in watching monitors that other grads didn't. I interviewed with them but I didn't have the experience. From there I just bugged them every three months or so. Finally, the recruiter had an ICU position come up and she called me because I had kept in touch, because she knew me." Jen suggests keeping in touch with the recruiters at desired locations, introducing yourself with a letter or by getting their names and calling them, and then making sure they remember that you are waiting for them. "Part of it is just luck; if they need you when you are looking, you might luck into something that you'd be waiting forever for otherwise."

> **//Right out of school I started knocking on doors . . . Finally, the recruiter had an ICU position come up and she called me because I had kept in touch, because she knew me."**

The most obvious place to look for a nursing job is in a hospital. Nurses also are needed in retirement communities, in government facilities, in schools, and in private practices. In fact, nursing in hospitals is not expected to grow as fast as other aspects of nursing, due to rising costs and a general trend away from inpatient care. The slack caused by fewer available hospital jobs will be taken up by increased opportunities in newer fields. Insurance companies now hire registered nurses to assist in case management and to ensure that insured patients are getting the correct kind of care from their health care providers. One of the fastest-growing fields in nursing is home health care. Nurses who care for people on a part-time basis in their homes are in great demand for a variety of reasons. Technology has enabled many people to live free of health care institutions, but these people may still require assistance with some of their treatments.

Many surgical centers and emergency medical centers are taking the place of hospital emergency rooms. This will provide work for nurses who require a flexible schedule but who do not wish to work in a hospital. The number of older people with functional disabilities is growing, and jobs will be available in long-term care facilities for specialized conditions such as Alzheimer's disease.

Registered nurses should look in local papers and on the Internet for positions, in addition to contacting preferred employers to ask what they may have available. Knowing where you would like to work, achieving educational credits in that field, and making sure those in charge of hiring know you are available are the key steps to finding a desirable nursing position.

WHERE CAN I GO FROM HERE?

Experienced registered nurses can advance in many ways. Those who want challenges beyond direct patient care may become teachers or administrators. Others continue their education and become clinical nurse specialists, nurse practitioners, certified nurse-midwives, or nurse anesthetists. Master's degrees and doctorates are required for many of these positions.

Related Jobs

Audiologists

Dietitians

Nutritionists

Occupational therapists

Paramedics

Pharmacists

Physical therapists

Physicians' assistants

Recreational therapists

Respiratory therapists

Speech-language pathologists

WHAT ARE SOME RELATED JOBS?

The U.S. Department of Labor classifies registered nurses with people in the "Health Assessment and Treating Occupations," a subcategory of the much broader "Professional Speciality Occupations" field. Also under the "Health Assessment and Treating Occupations" heading are dietitians and nutritionists, pharmacists, paramedics, occupational therapists, physical therapists, recreational therapists, respiratory therapists, physicians' assistants, audiologists, and speech-language pathologists.

WHAT ARE THE SALARY RANGES?

Salaries can range from $20,000 to $40,000 to $55,000 per year, depending on the level of responsibility, the length of time spent working in one institution,

WHAT ARE THE SALARY RANGES?, CONTINUED

experience, training received, and educational degrees earned. In 1996, the median weekly earnings of full-time salaried registed nurses were $697. The middle 50 percent earned between $571 and $868. The lowest 10 percent earned less than $415, while the top 10 percent earned more than $1,039 per week. According to the Buck Survey conducted by the American Health Care Association, staff RNs in chain nursing homes had median hourly earnings of $15.85 in 1996. The middle 50 percent earned between $14.03 and $17.73.

Most health care employers provide a good benefits plan for their workers, as well as flexible work schedules, child care, and bonuses. Educational incentives take the form of in-house training and tuition reimbursement, which can enable nurses to increase their skills and potential for advancement at no or little cost to themselves.

WHAT IS THE JOB OUTLOOK?

As with most health care fields, nursing is expected to grow faster than average in the next ten to fifteen years. As the cost for medical specialists skyrockets, more general health care practitioners will be in demand for the services that they can provide at less cost. Nurse practitioners, for example, can diagnose, treat, and manage uncomplicated health problems.

Technological advances in patient care and the health care needs of an aging population have created a demand for skilled nurses in many areas. Ambulatory, home health, and outpatient care are expected to provide the most employment opportunities, while need for nurses in hospitals will grow less rapidly. Registered nurses will be in high demand in nursing homes and in facilities that care for critically and terminally ill patients.

There are also many part-time job openings for nurses who do not want a full-time position.

Staying aware of trends in health care will give prospective nurses a good idea of the job market for their skills. Trade journals, association membership materials, and health-care laws all discuss the course that health care is taking today, and are a valuable source of information for predicting where the future demand in nursing will be.

Surgical Nurse

SUMMARY

DEFINITION
Surgical nurses *care for patients before, during, and after surgical procedures. From preoperative assessment to assisting the surgical team to postoperative evaluation, the surgical nurse uses specific medical knowledge and technical skills to provide patient care.*

ALTERNATIVE JOB TITLES
Circulating nurse
Medical surgical nurse
Operating room nurse
Peri-operative nurse
Scrub nurse

SALARY RANGE
$25,000 to $35,000 to $45,000+

EDUCATIONAL REQUIREMENTS
Bachelor of Science in Nursing degree; completion of a post graduate operating room course of study or hospital in-service program

CERTIFICATION OR LICENSING
Required

EMPLOYMENT OUTLOOK
Much faster than the average

HIGH SCHOOL SUBJECTS
Anatomy and Physiology
Biology
Chemistry
Health

PERSONAL INTERESTS
Exercise/Personal Fitness
Helping people: physical health/medicine
Science
Volunteering

He wasn't breathing! . . . The panic showed clearly on the elderly patient's face. The surgically created hole in his throat had not healed yet from his earlier operation, so it closed immediately after he coughed the breathing tube out. Cecil King, a surgical nurse, had assisted in the operation and now his routine postoperative visit turned into an emergency situation. In what seemed like hours, but was only minutes, Cecil grabbed a spare breathing tube and quickly worked the hole open and inserted the tube. The patient's breathing was restored and Cecil sighed with relief. Obviously, surgical nursing is much more than handing a scalpel to a surgeon.

WHAT DOES A SURGICAL NURSE DO?

When most people think of nurses, the image of a surgical nurse handing an instrument to a surgeon is probably what comes to mind. Surgical nurses assist surgeons during operations ranging from a tonsillectomy to open heart surgery. Surgical nurses work in the operating rooms of hospitals, both large and small. Some surgical nurses may also work at outpatient surgical facilities. Anywhere you find a surgeon performing an operation, you'll also find a surgical nurse.

WHAT DOES A SURGICAL NURSE DO?, CONTINUED

Although surgical nurses are often called *operating room nurses,* or *OR nurses,* there is a distinction between operating room nurses and surgical nurses. There is only one kind of surgical nurse—the nurse assisting the surgeon. However, there are two kinds of OR nurses—the *circulating nurse* and the *scrub nurse.* Scrub nurse is just another name for surgical nurse. On the other hand, the circulating nurse is a non-sterile member of the surgical staff. This nurse "circulates" through many operating rooms to take samples to the pathology lab and bring the results back to the surgeon. The circulating nurse acts as a liaison between the surgical team and the rest of the hospital during and after an operation. Unlike the scrub nurse (surgical nurse), the circulating nurse is not in the room during the actual surgery.

Lingo to Learn

Allograft: *A specific surgery in which diseased tissue or organs are replaced with healthy tissue or bones from a living donor or a cadaver.*

Ambulatory care: *Surgical care for patients in outpatient settings with short recovery times.*

Arthroscopic surgery: *Outpatient surgery using small instruments and incisions.*

Clinical surgical nurse specialist: *A nurse who has a graduate level education and is an expert in a surgical specialty.*

The duties of a surgical nurse begin long before the patient is wheeled into the operating room and continue long after the operation is over. Through all aspects of the job, the surgical nurse has to remain observant and continually assess the patient. High-stress situations call for the surgical nurse to be calm and cool while meeting the needs of both the surgical team and the patient. The duties of the surgical nurse can be divided into three areas, although all of the areas overlap and work together: preoperative (before the operation), operative (during the operation), and postoperative (after the operation).

Before surgery, the surgical nurse must prepare a patient physically, emotionally, and mentally for the upcoming surgical procedure. First, the surgical nurse assesses the patient's current state. Is the patient showing signs of stress? Is he or she in any physical pain? Does the patient have enough information about the procedure to help with any anxiety or fear? After assessing the patient, the surgical nurse may explain the upcoming surgery in more detail, take steps to alleviate stress, and measure the patient's vital processes (heart rate, blood pressure, and so on). Another major responsibility is communicating to the family of the patient as much information as possible about the nature of the surgery, its expected length, predicted results, and usual outcomes. Although the surgeon usually describes her primary goal for the surgery and the method she'll be using to the patient's family, surgical nurses are often able to give more detailed information about the patient's well-being.

The surgical nurse may also be responsible for preparing the operating room for the surgery, including choosing and sterilizing the correct instruments and tools, setting up medical machinery, and keeping accurate count of the tools that will be used in the procedure.

During surgery, the surgical nurse's primary duty is to assist the surgeons in the operating room. The surgical nurse must anticipate the needs of the surgical team and react to any changes in the patient's physical state. Since all surgery has a certain amount of risk, operations must be performed as quickly as possible. Because of this, surgical nurses must be familiar with many different procedures and the instruments and tools that are used to perform them. During the operation, the surgical nurse must be prepared to act on the surgeon's instructions.

After the operation, the surgical nurse continues to evaluate the patient, but at this stage the questions are a little different. How is the patient responding to the surgery? Is the medication relieving any postoperative pain the patient may have? Is the patient recovering as expected? Also, the surgical nurse relays the pertinent information concerning the surgery and its results to the patient's family. The surgical nurse will visit the patient periodically to monitor his or her progress and administer any medications prescribed by the surgeon or physician.

WHAT IS IT LIKE TO BE A SURGICAL NURSE?

As assistant nurse manager of the Main Operating Rooms at the University of Washington Medical Center in Seattle, Cecil King thinks he has made his last career stop. "Right now, with the changing climate of health care, people like myself set their own limits," Cecil explains. "There are such vast opportunities for one willing to take risks, be visionary, and not set limitations on possibilities."

It's no wonder that Cecil finds great satisfaction as a part of the surgical medical team. Surgical nursing is an exciting, fast-paced career that constantly challenges a nurse's ability to cope under pressure. When the patient's loss of his breathing tube required quick and decisive action by Cecil (described in the introduction to this article), he described it as "the longest and scariest couple of minutes of my life." But the rewards of helping to save a man's life far outweigh even the most frightening situations.

Surgical nurses usually work an extended day to evening shift since most surgeries are scheduled during that time. Common shifts include 1:00 PM to 9:30 PM, 6:30 AM to 3:00 PM, and so on. Most surgical nurses are also on call, so if an emergency situation arises or the staff is short on a given day, a surgical nurse can be called in to work. Most nurses dislike that aspect of the job and say it is the most difficult part of being a surgical nurse.

Long hours are often the norm for surgical nurses as well. Regular shifts plus emergency surgeries can add up to a lot of high-stress work and very little sleep. "Having to come in for an emergency at 2:00 in the morning and then having to be ready for my regular shift at 7:00 that same morning gets a little tough," says Bonnie Deitz, an operating room manager. Cecil agrees, "The down side to surgical nursing is always being on call."

Once on the job, a nursing manager assigns patients to the surgical nurse. Preoperative care begins as soon as a patient is scheduled for surgery. The surgical nurse meets with the patient right away to prepare him or her for the operation. Depending on the complexity of the operation, the surgical nurse will begin measuring the patient's vital functions to determine if he or she is at the physical level needed for the operation. Many times, the patient may not be ready and the operation is postponed. The surgical nurse must make this judgment call and alert the surgeon, who then decides if the patient is strong enough to go through with the procedure.

Also during this time the surgical nurse will meet with the family to discuss exactly what will be happening to the patient during the operation. The surgical nurse also discusses the patient's physical status with the surgeon. "In surgical nursing, you must always be able to work as part of a team and be able to communicate with other nurses and surgeons as well as the patients and their families," explains Bonnie.

As the patient is taken into surgery, the surgical nurse has already prepared the operating room for maximum efficiency. The surgical nurse sterilizes and sets out all the necessary tools and prepares the machinery for use during the operation. Any special items requested by the surgical team are taken care of by the surgical nurse. No matter what type of operation is being performed, the surgical nurse assists the surgeon with whatever he or she may need. First, the surgical nurse is at the operating table handing proper instruments to the surgeon. Secondly, the surgical nurse constantly monitors the patient as the operation proceeds.

In the recovery room, the focus shifts to making sure the patient is recuperating well. The surgical nurse watches for signs that the procedure was or was not successful. Any and all variations are reported to the attending physician or surgeon.

Every surgery is different because every patient has different needs. With all the different types of surgery and different methods surgeons use, the surgical nurse must keep abreast of all kinds of technical information. "It's hard to know one particular area very well, so instead I'm a generalist," Cecil explains. "I am now challenged to become an expert generalist in my profession."

Every day, surgical nurses are met with new challenges and come up with new ways to meet them. "The thing I most enjoy about being a surgical nurse is that each day is always different, and because of that you develop a close working relationship with the other nurses and surgeons," explains Bonnie.

HAVE I GOT WHAT IT TAKES TO BE A SURGICAL NURSE?

"Just today I got a phone call that they are looking for another person for a case on Sunday morning. I may have to change all of my plans to come in to work," said Bonnie as she described the ups and downs of being "on call." Most nurses describe the odd hours as the most demanding part of their job. Never knowing when they will have to drop what they are doing and go into a high-stress situation, surgical nurses are called upon to be very flexible. To be a surgical nurse, you have to be willing to put your life on hold sometimes. "The hours can vary and be demanding; one needs emotional and physical stamina," Cecil advises.

To be a successful surgical nurse, you should:

Have compassion and be willing to put your patient's needs first

Be flexible to work odd hours and be on call

Be alert and constantly aware of the patients under your care

Be able to cope with the physical and mental demands of emergency situations

Follow instructions completely and pay attention to detail

Relate well to people and have strong communication skills

Surgical nurses deal with situations ranging from minor surgery to life-and-death surgical procedures. As a part of a surgical team, you must be able to deal with the pressure that comes with holding a person's life in your hands. As a surgical nurse, you must be able to react quickly to emergencies by drawing on your technical knowledge and experience. Cecil feels a person who is best suited for surgical nursing "must like the sciences and care about people. Nursing is an art and science of caring and interfacing for patients when they cannot speak or act for themselves."

If you get woozy at the sight of blood, this is probably not the best career choice for you. But, if you are fascinated by the workings of the human body or intrigued by how modern medical procedures can prolong life, this may be your best bet. This isn't a profession for people who want a nine-to-five job that they can leave behind when they get home. Surgical nursing is a field for people who want to make a difference for other people and are willing to give a large portion of their own lives to do so.

HOW DO I BECOME A SURGICAL NURSE?

EDUCATION

High School

In all states you must graduate from a nursing program and then be certified. To enter a nursing program, you must have a high school degree. As a high school student, you should take as many science, biology, health, and mathematics classes as you can. And, because communication skills are so important in the nursing field as a whole and surgical nursing in particular, you should also take speech and English classes.

Cecil King advises high school students to take as many college preparatory classes as they can and computer classes as well. He also recommends taking first aid courses as provided by your school or other agencies. "I studied college prep and all the sciences offered, joined the science club, was a lifeguard, and read all the time," Cecil explains. "Some high schools have future nurses clubs that work with school nurses to help students explore careers in nursing."

On the practical side, you can gain a lot of hands-on experience through volunteering or getting a part-time job in a hospital. Bonnie Deitz says her experience as a volunteer candy striper "allowed me to become familiar with a hospital environment."

As a surgical nurse looking back, Cecil advises, "Take your education very seriously and demand to get the best education you can. Use every learning resource available to you. If you are truly interested in nursing, seek out nurses to talk to and maybe share time with them on the job."

Postsecondary Training

Though there are three ways to continue your education in general nursing—the baccalaureate program, the associate degree program, and the hospital diploma program—the baccalaureate program is the level of education necessary to pursue surgical nursing. The baccalaureate program leads to a bachelor of science in nursing (BSN) degree and usually takes four years to complete at most colleges and universities. While you can start out earning the associate's degree or the hospital diploma, you will have to eventually earn a BSN degree to be qualified for surgical nursing. Bonnie illustrates this point very well with her own experience, "If I could go back and do things differently, I would have gotten my degree (BSN) right away. But, when I went to school, the norm was a diploma program. We took all the same classes as offered in college, but because they were taught at the nursing school and not at the college, credits were not given."

// Take your education very seriously and demand to get the best education you can. Use every learning resource available to you. If you are truly interested in nursing, seek out nurses to talk to and maybe share time with them on the job."

Over six hundred colleges and universities in the United States offer the BSN degree. You'll take classes in nursing theory, humanities, sciences, human growth and development, and so on. You'll also take part in clinical experience programs at hospitals and other health care facilities in the last two years of your degree program. Bonnie recommends that anyone entering college today for a nursing career should "take any extra courses offered for the specific specialty you are interested in. And always remember that nothing is permanent and new opportunities will present themselves."

After earning a BSN degree, you must also enroll in a formal, postgraduate operating room course or participate in a hospital in-service program that focuses on the development of the necessary skills and techniques of surgical nursing.

Cecil offers this advice, "Go to one of the top ten schools of nursing and pursue your BSN. While you're there, pursue clinical experience and take electives in peri-operative nursing."

CERTIFICATION OR LICENSING

After getting your BSN degree, you must then spend two years gaining work experience in surgical nursing before you are eligible to become certified. After

HOW DO I BECOME A . . . ?, CONTINUED

you have two years of experience, you can take the exam to become a certified nurse: operating room (CNOR). The exam is given on a computer through the National Certification Board: Perioperative Nursing, Inc. The exam will measure your expert peri-operative nursing knowledge.

Once you receive certification, you are certified for five years. To renew, you can either earn 150 hours of continuing education over the five-year period or take the exam again. "I think nurses should seek certification in their specialty as a measure of excellence for the public to see," Cecil says.

INTERNSHIPS AND VOLUNTEERSHIPS

As part of your BSN degree, you will be required to complete several nursing internships or clinicals. Usually these clinicals are set up through the college or university to be completed at a hospital or other health care facility.

Volunteering is an excellent way to gain experience and build up your resume. Contact hospitals, nursing homes, and other health care facilities to find out about volunteering (or maybe even part-time employment) as a nurse's aide or office helper. Not only will you learn while doing, you may also make valuable contacts that can be helpful in getting a job later in your career.

WHO WILL HIRE ME?

Cecil began his nursing training in the Navy Hospital Corpsman School as a Navy hospital corpsman/operating room technician. During his time in the Navy, Cecil discovered how much he enjoyed nursing, so after leaving the Service, he enrolled at the University of Maryland. "Being an OR tech in the Navy before going to nursing school was a great way for me to start my career," Cecil said. Cecil worked as an OR technician at the R. Adams Cowley Shock Trauma Center at the University of Maryland. "My work at the R. Adams Center allowed me to easily move into a staff nurse position on the inpatient unit of the center as a new graduate," Cecil explains.

Nursing graduates often follow this pattern of seeking employment in the same hospital or health care facility in which they completed their clinical work. It's important to select a college or university that has a strong clinical program. The best programs will be affiliated with a hospital or outpatient facility so that nursing students can work during their schooling to fulfill experience requirements.

The two major employment areas for surgical nurses are hospitals and ambulatory surgery centers (outpatient surgery centers). Hospitals in the larger cities usually employ many surgical nurses to meet the needs of the high number of patients and surgeries that are necessary. Outpatient surgery is on the rise due to hospitals trying to cut costs by releasing patients earlier and moving many surgical procedures that were once inpatient to outpatient status. Although hospitals employ the most nurses overall, nursing jobs in outpatient facilities are growing every year. The United States Bureau of Labor Statistics states that jobs in outpatient facilities will grow by 81 percent by the year 2005. There are about 6,000 hospitals in the U.S. today and ambulatory care centers are everywhere. The Veterans Affairs health care system itself has over 170 hospitals and 200 clinics throughout the country. In other words, you shouldn't have to look very far to find a health care facility with which you can seek employment.

Excerpt from the Nurses' Code of Ethics

1. To conserve life, alleviate suffering and promote health.

2. To give nursing care that is not influenced or altered by the personality of the patient, race, social status, religion, or any other external factor.

3. To maintain high standards of ethics in personal life and to practice good citizenship.

4. To keep up-to-date with current nursing practice to be adequately prepared to give the best possible care to the patient.

5. To carry out orders with the greatest skill possible.

Source: The American Nurses Association Code of Ethics

The first place a new graduate should visit when looking for a nursing position is the career services office at the college or university he or she has attended. They should be able to provide leads and contact information, and sometimes they will set up interviews immediately with certain health care facilities. Often the places a nursing student worked during clinical experience programs for college are the best starting points for employment. Job seekers can also go the traditional route by checking the employment advertising in the newspaper. Nursing magazines such as *American Nurse, Nursing, RN,* and the *Ambulatory Nursing Journal* can usually be found in the larger libraries and often contain advertisements for open positions.

The following associations publish materials that contain job listings or hospital listings: American Hospital Association, American Medical Association, American Nurses Association, Association of Operating Room Nurses, and the National Student Nurses Association. You'll find contact information for these associations at the end of this book.

The Internet also provides a wealth of employment listings that are updated daily. Job seekers should search the Internet with keywords such as "nursing and employment," "nursing and jobs," and "nursing and career." Check out the Surf the Web chapter at the end of this book, too.

WHERE CAN I GO FROM HERE?

After becoming an OR staff nurse at the Shock Trauma Center at the University of Maryland, Cecil advanced in this same field as an assistant nurse manager of the Main OR for the University of Washington Medical Center in Seattle. Cecil is still involved in the surgical care of patients, but he is now a clinical perioperative specialist for the operating room. This clinical leadership position allows Cecil to schedule his own hours to meet the needs of the OR. He continued his education and is close to earning his master's degree in nursing.

Cecil's advancement within the surgical nursing field places him in a leadership position in charge of other staff nurses. He spends a lot of his time answering clinical questions and concerns. Cecil also works on developing standards of practice and various projects in research and development around clinical issues. Along with all of that, he is still often needed to staff evening surgeries and give direct patient care. As a part of this leadership role, he is on call twenty-four hours a day and acts as a troubleshooter for the surgical nursing staff. Cecil describes the sub-roles of his work as "leading, managing, consulting, researching, and educating."

Advancement Possibilities

Clinical surgical nurse specialists supervise and guide surgical nurses through daily routines. Clinical nurse specialists also conduct research and develop nursing techniques.

Nurse practitioners perform many tasks without supervision that are usually reserved for physicians, such as treating common ailments, administering medications, and examining patients.

Nurse managers for operating rooms coordinate and oversee nursing areas of the surgical unit. Nurse managers assist head nurses and their staff with difficult surgical situations.

Nursing instructors give classroom instruction for the nursing staff and supervise nurses on duty in hospital units.

Although advancement in the surgical nursing field doesn't have to follow exactly the same path as Cecil's, a nurse seeking to advance must follow many of the same steps. It's important to continue to educate yourself if you want to move up to higher-skilled, more responsible positions. A master's degree and then a doctorate are both steps that may need to be completed for certain positions. You may want to become a clinical nurse specialist in the medical-surgical area or perhaps you'll shift laterally to become a clinical nurse specialist in a slightly different area. Whatever your goal, more education and ongoing experience is the key. You may even decide to become your own boss as a nurse practitioner.

There is also a great deal of advancement opportunity on the business side of nursing. You can use your experience and knowledge to manage an ambulatory care center. You may even advance to high-level management jobs within a hospital or health organization. The opportunities are really wide open. In fact, Cecil feels that most nurses with ongoing education and experience will be able to set their own limits regarding advancement in the field of nursing.

WHAT ARE SOME RELATED JOBS?

Most emergency, critical care, and operative nursing jobs have similarities with surgical nursing. Any nursing position where care of the patient has several stages and includes pressure-intensive situations is close to the requirements for surgical nursing.

Related Jobs

Clinical nurse specialists

Critical care nurses

Emergency room nurses

Nurse anesthetists

Nurse-midwives

Nurse practitioners

Operating room technicians

Transplant nurses

The U.S. Department of Labor classifies surgical nurses under the heading Registered Nurses (DOT) and Nursing (GOE). Also under this heading are people who provide care for patients, assist physicians and other nurses, administer medical care according to physician instructions, perform emergency medical care, examine patients, maintain patient histories, evaluate patients, and communicate with the families of patients.

WHAT ARE THE SALARY RANGES?

Salary ranges for surgical nurses often depend on what region of the country they are working in and the level of education and experience attained. Generally, surgical nursing positions in the West pay the highest, followed by the East Coast, and then the middle South. Surgical nurses usually average around $30,000 per year. The low side is about $25,000 and the high side is $45,000 and above. The University of Texas Medical Branch survey listed staff nurses (RNs) at about $33,000 and clinical nurse specialists at an average salary of about $47,000. Similarly, the Kellogg School of Management survey lists $35,000 as the average annual salary for a staff OR nurse.

Hospitals usually have very attractive benefits packages to go along with the yearly salary. Often this includes tuition reimbursement to help you further your education while you work. If you work for a government hospital, you will get state employee benefits which are usually very comprehensive.

WHAT IS THE JOB OUTLOOK?

The job outlook for surgical nursing, and nursing in general for that matter, is excellent and shows no sign of changing in the near future. Nursing is expected to grow faster than the average for all occupations in the United States through the year 2006. While the outlook for general nurses is excellent, its employment focus is shifting from hospitals to outpatient care. This is not necessarily true for surgical nurses. Although hospitals are trying to cut costs by moving patients out of the hospital more quickly and by making more operations outpatient, this does not diminish the need for surgical nurses. Whether in the hospital setting or in an ambulatory care setting, surgical nurses continue to be in high demand.

Another factor that is affecting nursing is the growth of the segment of the American population that is sixty-five and over. As this elderly population grows and as people live longer, there is more of a chance that body organs and systems will wear out, creating a need for surgical care. Surgical nurses will continue to be in high demand as the population ages.

The increasing need for surgical care will also increase the number of surgeries performed in ambulatory care settings. Surgical nurses with specific skills and techniques will be in high demand to meet the ambulatory care needs.

Hospitals may try to offset costs by using more part-time nurses. Currently, one-fourth to one-third of all nurses work on a part-time schedule. This may be less of a factor for surgical nurses because of their education and experience levels.

What Can I Do Right Now

Nursing

?

Get Involved

Now that you've read about different careers in nursing, what do you think is the most important characteristic a prospective nurse should have? If you think it's the desire to help others, then you're developing a good understanding of this profession. The fact is that nursing, above all else, is about caring for other people, so nurses must put their patients first. It's certainly true that nurses find their work intellectually stimulating, challenging, exciting, and personally fulfilling—but they find their ultimate reward in the care and comfort they give to others.

After this desire to help, what do you suppose is the next most important characteristic of a prospective nurse? Is it academic ability? Practical nursing skills? Bedside manner? Personal maturity? Dedication to the work even under difficult circumstances? You probably know by now that *all* of these things are equally important. If you're not quite convinced of that, consider a nursing student who gets straight A's in her classes but can't calm a nervous patient down to give him his medication. Or consider a nursing student who gets along beautifully with all of the patients he works with but is never on time to feed them or bathe them. They both may have the desire to serve and other skills besides, but their behavior may prove harmful to their patients—and it certainly won't endear them to prospective employers.

We can conclude that nurses must be strong in three general areas, broadly defined as academic ability, practical skill, and personal character. This may seem a bit overwhelming, but you can easily start to evaluate and improve your proficiency in these areas right now, while you are still in high school. This section will introduce you to some of the many ways in which you can test your aptitude for nursing and begin to prepare for a nursing career.

ACADEMIC ABILITY

Academic ability is undoubtedly the area you're most familiar with, since you spend at least nine months out of the year working on it! If you want to be a nurse, you simply must be confident of your abilities in biology, chemistry, composition, mathematics, and the other subjects that are essential to the profession. That's not to say that you must enjoy all these subjects and earn top grades in them, but you must be comfortable with each one. If you need to improve in one or more of these subjects—and most people have plenty of room for improvement—start now by really applying yourself and asking your teachers for advice and assistance. Good performances in high school classes will not only aid your nursing school applications, they'll also make your college classes much more manageable.

PRACTICAL SKILL

Practical skills are those that are specific to nursing: giving a patient an injection, assisting a physician, comforting an accident victim. Naturally, you will learn and practice these skills in college, but you can start working on some of them while you're still in high school. Doing so will give you a real advantage and added confidence in nursing school, and will also give you the chance to explore the profession before making a commitment to it. You may be able to learn enough right now to start thinking about pursuing a nursing specialty such as pediatrics or midwifery. Then, too, you may learn that you are not as well suited to the profession as you thought. If you feel faint at the sight of blood or constantly lose your patience with those who are ill and not in good humor, don't you want to know this before you invest time and money in nurse's training?

PERSONAL QUALITIES

The personal character traits needed for nursing are not as easy to quantify as the other skills and abilities. Nurses are, of course, unique individuals with different likes, dislikes, backgrounds, aspirations, and qualities. But they do share a profound sense of dedication, responsibility, and maturity. While these characteristics are important to virtually every profession, they are absolutely vital to nursing, where the health and well-being of others is on the line. Again, you don't have to wait until you're a full-time nursing student to put your character to the test. You can take advantage of many opportunities right now to examine and improve upon your sense of responsibility and maturity. In fact, you'll probably find that almost all of the opportunities mentioned below require a bit more dedication and mature behavior than most of the situations you've been in before.

PREPARING FOR NURSING: ACADEMIC ABILITY

As we've said, preparing academically for a nursing career is something you're already doing five days a week for the better part of the year. So why would you want to work on biology or chemistry over the summer as well? There are a number of reasons. If you need to improve on certain subjects, summer gives you the extra time you need to do so. If you're already doing well in school, use and expand your knowledge during the summertime instead of slowly forgetting what you've learned—or try a subject, perhaps anatomy or nutrition, that your home school doesn't offer. And since many summer study opportunities are offered by colleges and universities around the country, they give you the chance to experience college-level classes and campus life before you're even out of high school.

Below is a sampling of the academic camps and study programs that are available. Remember that we don't endorse any of these programs, but we do want you to check them out for yourself. And be sure to check around your own area or at your preferred colleges to see what's available there.

THE PROGRAMS

ADVANCED BIOLOGICAL SCIENCES INSTITUTE

Wright State University (WSU) offers a wide selection of Pre-College Programs every July for high school students. If you are a rising junior or senior who is considering a nursing career, WSU has a special study option for you. The Advanced Biological Sciences Institute is a week and a half of instruction and exploration under the guidance of WSU's School of Medicine and College of Sciences and Mathematics.

All participants join in seminars, workshops, and other activities in each of the following departments: anatomy, biochemistry, biological sciences, microbiology and immunology, and physiology and biophysics. Some dissection or examination of biological specimens may be included in the laboratory activities. This is a very selective program with only twenty-four spaces available. Applicants must have completed at least one high school course in biology and preferably one in chemistry as well. The application form must be submitted with a transcript and letter of recommendation by June. WSU awards college credit to those who successfully complete the program. The total cost for this residential program is about $1,100, all-inclusive except for transportation to and from Dayton, Ohio.

Wright State University also offers Pre-College Programs for junior high school students, but not a program comparable to the Advanced Biological Sciences Institute. Contact the WSU Office of Pre-College Programs for more information.

■ **Advanced Biological Sciences Institute**
Wright State University Pre-College Programs
163 Millett Hall, 3640 Colonel Glenn Highway
Dayton, OH 45435-0001
Tel: 937-775-3135
Fax: 937-775-4883

AMERICAN COLLEGIATE ADVENTURES

American Collegiate Adventures (ACA) offers high school students the chance to experience and prepare for college during summer vacation. Adventures are based at Arizona State University in Tempe and the University of Wisconsin in Madison; they vary in length from three to six weeks. Participants attend college-level courses taught by university faculty during the week (for college credit or enrichment) and visit regional colleges and recreation sites over the weekend. All students live in comfortable en suite accommodations, just down the hall from an ACA resident staff member. Courses vary but usually include such basics as "Introduction to Biology" and "Introduction to Chemistry"— perfect for those planning to pursue a degree in nursing. Contact American Collegiate Adventures for the current course listings, prices, and application procedures.

■ **American Collegiate Adventures**
666 Dundee Road
Suite 803
Northbrook, IL 60062
Tel: 800-509-SUMR or 847-509-9900
Fax: 847-509-9908
Email: ACASUMR@aol.com

BENJAMIN E. MAYS SCHOLARS IN BIOLOGY PROGRAM

Bates University hosts the Benjamin E. Mays Scholars in Biology Program for rising juniors and seniors. This residential program runs for nearly two weeks in July, during which students complete five two-day units on various aspects of college-level biology. The exact topics of the units change each year, but those offered in 1997 included The Biology of DNA, Biochemistry of Proteins and Carbohydrates, and Human and Animal Nerve and Muscle Physiology. Those interested in the field of nursing may rest assured that virtually every aspect of human biology will figure prominently in their education and career. All units of the Scholars in Biology Program are taught by faculty from the Bates College departments of biology and chemistry. Participating students live in Bates College dormitories and are welcome to use such campus facilities as the indoor pool, tennis courts, and the Museum of Art. Applicants must submit a completed form, transcript, essay, and letter of evaluation from a teacher or principal by the end of April. Only about eighteen places are available each year, so admission is competitive. For an application and further information, contact the Director of Special Projects and Summer Programs.

Benjamin E. Mays Scholars in Biology Program
Office of Special Projects and Summer Programs
Bates College, 163 Wood Street
Lewiston, ME 04240-6016
Tel: 207-786-6077
Fax: 207-786-6025
Web: http://www.bates.edu

CHEMISTRY IS FUN! CAMP

Chemistry Is Fun! is one of several camps offered each summer by the Center for Chemical Education at Miami University of Ohio. Rising ninth- and tenth-graders are welcome to participate in this week-long program that explores the field of chemistry. During Chemistry is Fun!, you explore different aspects of the field and conduct your own chemistry experiments in one of Miami University's laboratories. Every nurse must have a solid understanding of chemistry, so it can be worthwhile to explore the subject in such a positive and enthusiastic setting. The camp lasts three hours a day for five days, generally a week in mid-July. It costs only about $75 and financial aid is available.

Note that this camp is usually held at the university's campus in Oxford, Ohio and not in Middletown; however, for specific details on this year's Chemistry Is Fun! Camp, contact the Middletown campus.

Chemistry Is Fun! Camp
Miami University Middletown
4200 East University Boulevard
Middletown, OH 45042
Tel: 513-727-3269

CORNELL UNIVERSITY SUMMER COLLEGE

Rising and graduating seniors with an interest in nursing are invited to apply to Cornell University's Summer College, where you can participate in the Exploration in Biological Research and the Health Professions. Students at the six-week, residential Summer College choose two regular university courses in conjunction with an area of career exploration. The explorations take place three afternoons per week and involve field trips, discussions, and meetings with professionals employed in the field. Those students who select the Exploration in Biological Research and the Health Professions meet with research scientists, physicians, and practitioners in allied health fields, and tour laboratories and other facilities related to your special interests, including obstetrics, physical therapy, and nursing. Your two courses can be in any areas—from economics to the arts—but Cornell recommends that students in this exploration take one biology course and one writing course. Full college credit will be awarded by Cornell University upon successful completion of the courses (no credit is given for the explorations). Participants should expect a challenging curriculum and mature environment very different from high school; these, of course, are two of the attractions of Cornell University's Summer College. The cost of this program is about $3,500 for tuition and $1,500 for room and board; some financial aid is available.

Interested students should submit the application form and fee, current transcript with standardized test scores, and a letter of recommendation by the beginning of May. Those applying for financial aid must submit their materials by the beginning of April. For further information, including a catalogue of courses and an application form, contact the Director of the Summer College.

Cornell University Summer College
B20 Day Hall
Ithaca, NY 14853-2801
Tel: 607-255-6203
Fax: 607-255-9697
Web: http://www.sce.cornell.edu/SC/
Email: sc@sce.cornell.edu

MEDCAMP

Arizona high school students in their sophomore year might have the opportunity to attend MedCamp during their summer vacation. The University of Arizona Health Sciences Center (AHSC) has sponsored this free, three-day career camp every July since 1992. High schools around the state nominate one boy and one girl for the program; the nominees may then submit an application and essay, by which the final participants are selected. If you are chosen to attend MedCamp, you will then explore medical careers while living on the University of Arizona campus under the supervision of medical students. During the day, there are classes, laboratory experiences, hospital tours, and opportunities to speak with and watch health care professionals at work. You leave with a better overall understanding of the health care industry and information on specific careers such as nursing, physical and occupational therapy, and pharmacy. If you are interested in attending MedCamp, discuss it with your science teacher, who should receive nomination forms from the AHSC.

■ **Medcamp**
University of Arizona Health Sciences Center
Office of Public Affairs, PO Box 245095
Tucson, AZ 85724-5095
Tel: 520-626-7301

PRE-COLLEGE PROGRAM AT JOHNS HOPKINS

Johns Hopkins University welcomes academically talented high school students to its summertime Pre-College Program. Participants in this program live on Hopkins' Homewood campus for five weeks beginning in early July. They pursue one of six programs leading to college credit; those interested in nursing should strongly consider the program Medical Science: Exploring the Options. In the medical science program, students take two college-level courses. The first is "Introduction to Biological Molecules," which surveys the important structures and functions of macromolecules involved in biological processes. For your second course, you may choose either "Modern Medicine: A Historical Introduction" or "Anthropology of Health and Medical Science." The former is a scientific and historical look at medicine from the Renaissance to today; the latter examines medicine in its cultural and social contexts. Coursework is supplemented with presentations by research scientists, laboratory tours, and visits to the famous Johns Hopkins Hospital and Medical School. All participants in the Pre-College Program also attend workshops on college admissions, time management, and diversity. The cost of the program is around $4,000, including tuition, room, board, workshops, field trips, and other scheduled extracurricular activities. Students who live in the greater Baltimore area have the option of commuting; they pay about $2,500 for all of the other expenses. Contact the Office of Summer Programs for financial aid information. As of July 1, applicants must be at least sixteen, have completed their sophomore, junior, or senior year, and have a minimum GPA of 3.0. By mid-April, they must submit an application form, essay, transcript, two recommendations, and a non-refundable application fee (rates vary by date of submission). For more information, including an application form, contact the Office of Summer Programs.

Pre-College Program
Johns Hopkins University
230 Mergenthaler Hall, 3400 North Charles Street
Baltimore, MD 21218-2685
Tel: 410-516-4548
Web: http://www.jhu.edu/~sumprog
Email: summer@jhu.edu

PRIME, INC.

PRIME is a nonprofit organization founded in 1973 and dedicated to "creating opportunities for minorities in mathematics and science-based professions." It runs various programs involving high school students in interesting math and science projects as well as career exploration. Some programs run during the school year, others during the summer, and there are specialized programs for students needing supplemental instruction. PRIME emphasizes nursing as a profession and not only offers preparation in the subjects basic to nursing studies and careers, but also helps interested participants visit hospitals and other medical facilities. There is no cost to students participating in any PRIME program as it is underwritten by private donors and corporate sponsors. If you think PRIME may be able to help you reach your goals, speak to a science teacher or guidance counselor about getting involved. Middle school students can also participate in many of PRIME's programs.

PRIME, Inc.
7790 Dungan Road
Philadelphia, PA 19111
Tel: 215-697-8700
Fax: 215-697-8701

PROJECT GAIN (GET AHEAD IN NURSING) CAMP

In conjunction with its Get Ahead in Nursing (GAIN) program, the School of Nursing at Southern Illinois University at Edwardsville (SIUE) offers a six-week Summer Nurse Camp. Most participants have spent the previous school year as active members of GAIN clubs, which focus on helping disadvantaged students to successfully pursue degrees in nursing. All students must live in the

Edwardsville area, as the camp is not residential and camp transportation only runs to pickup points at local high schools. Participants are divided into three levels at the Summer Nurse Camp, but all pursue a rigorous, highly structured course of experiential study. All students take part in laboratory activities and practice taking vital signs and administering basic First Aid and CPR. First-year participants (grouped as Level I) take field trips to clinical facilities while returning students (Level II) actually serve in such a facility two days each week. Those who are spending their third year at the Summer Nurse Camp (Level III) serve four days per week in a clinical setting and may be eligible to participate in the Basic Nurse Assistant Program to become Certified Nurse Aides. Students at all levels are taught and supervised by SIUE faculty and nursing professionals from area hospitals. The cost of the program is only about $50, which covers such expenses as a camp t-shirt, name badge, and field trips. For more information about Project GAIN and how you can participate in its Summer Nurse Camp, contact the SIUE School of Nursing.

> ■**Project GAIN (Get Ahead in Nursing) Summer Camp**
> Southern Illinois University at Edwardsville
> School of Nursing, Box 1066
> Edwardsville, IL 62026-1066
> Tel: 618-692-3956
> Fax: 618-692-3854

SECONDARY STUDENT TRAINING PROGRAM (SSTP) RESEARCH PARTICIPATION

The Secondary Student Training Program (SSTP) at the University of Iowa has enabled high school students to participate in scientific research projects since 1959. The SSTP runs for five weeks, from late June until the beginning of August. It is a residential program, with students living on campus and enjoying all the recreational facilities of the University of Iowa. Participants spend roughly forty hours per week in one of the laboratories on campus pursuing research with University faculty and staff. Research projects are available in many sciences, but students considering nursing careers might want to undertake research in anatomy, biochemistry, biology, pathology or pediatrics. Besides getting a head start on college courses, such research helps to familiarize you with the latest techniques and equipment for scientific inquiry, library research, and data analysis. You also attend seminars featuring researchers, writers, and philosophers addressing ethical issues, public policy concerns, and career choices. At the end of the SSTP, all participants present their research to a symposium of their peers and mentors. Clearly, this is a demanding program and only those students with proven mathematical and scientific abilities are accepted. Students who have completed the tenth, eleventh, or twelfth grade and who have at least a B average (3.0 GPA on a 4.0 scale) are eligible. The cost of the SSTP is roughly $1,700, which includes everything but spending money and transportation costs; some financial aid is available. For application materials and further information, contact the Secondary Student Training Program.

Secondary Student Training Program (SSTP) Research Participation
University of Iowa
323 Chemistry Building D
Iowa City, IA 52242-1294
Tel: 319-335-0040
Fax: 319-335-3802

SUMMER AT DELPHI

Whether you're trying to catch up or get ahead on a course, Summer at Delphi may offer the opportunity you need. The Delphian School is a private, nonsectarian day and residential school for students ages five to seventeen, but its summer session is open to students from other schools around the country. Delphi adheres to the educational philosophy of L. Ron Hubbard, who created innovative study methods and emphasized the responsibility of the individual for his or her own academic success. Many of the courses offered for high school students during Summer at Delphi are perfectly suited for those considering a nursing career; in 1997, they included "Anatomy and Physiology," "Basic First Aid," "Cell Biology," the "Circulatory System," and "Nutrition and Exercise." You can also work on such fundamentals as algebra, chemistry, and composition. Each course curriculum is personally tailored to your needs, so you are challenged but not held back or left behind by other students. All students, however, participate in computer training, service projects, and various trips and activities. You may enroll as a day or resident student, for a term of four, six, seven, or eight weeks.

Resident students can expect to pay from $2,600 to $3,600, depending on length of stay. Contact the Delphian School to discuss its educational philosophy and to determine if it is right for you.

Summer at Delphi
The Delphian School
20950 SW Rock Creek Road
Sheridan, OR 97378
Tel: 800-626-6610
Web: http://www.theschool.com
Email: newinqs@theschool.com

SUMMER NURSING CAMP

Research College of Nursing, in conjunction with Rockhurst College, offers a residential Summer Nursing Camp for one week in early June. This is open to rising juniors and seniors, though preference is given to seniors. Participants experience college-level courses in nursing concepts at Research College of Nursing and perform some laboratory work at Rockhurst College. During the camp, you explore the many different options available in professional nursing and consider nursing's central role in today's health care systems. You also spend a day shadowing a nurse at Research Medical Center. Campers live in the Research Student Village (adjacent to the Medical Center) where you have access to such recreational facilities as a gymnasium and outdoor pool. The camp counselor is a current nursing student. The cost of the Summer Nursing Camp is about $225, which includes room and board, recreation and instructional activities, and some equipment that is yours to keep. Applications are due in mid-May along with a health status form and recommendation from a guidance counselor. Acceptance is based largely on academic performance, particularly in math and science classes. For further details and application information, contact the Summer Nursing Camp in care of Rockhurst College.

Summer Nursing Camp
Rockhurst College
1100 Rockhurst Road
Kansas City, MO 64110-2561
Tel: 816-501-4100 or 800-842-6776

SUMMER SCIENCE AND MATH WORKSHOP

High school girls from the New York metropolitan area can apply to the Marymount College Summer Science and Math Workshop. The two-week residential workshop is designed to inspire rising sophomores, juniors, and seniors to continue studying math and science and to consider careers in those fields. Part of your time is spent on experiments in biology, chemistry, and physics, and on group projects in these and related subjects. Much of your remaining time is spent on career exploration. Health care is among the career fields explored during the course of the Summer Science and Math Workshop, but you will also have the opportunity to learn more about the financial, telecommunications, and environmental fields, among others. There are also field trips to laboratories and other facilities not usually open to high school students, and you will have the experience of living in college dormitories and using Marymount's own recreational facilities. The only cost to participants is a $100 materials fee (which may be covered by a scholarship, if necessary). The workshop usually runs from late June to early July; applications are usually due at the beginning of April, and there is an information session for you and your parents at the beginning of March. Contact the director if you would like to receive more information and an application form.

Summer Science and Math Workshop
Marymount College, #1173
100 Marymount Avenue
Tarrytown, NY 10591-3796
Tel: 914-332-8291
Fax: 914-631-8586

PREPARING FOR NURSING: PRACTICAL SKILL

You probably already know of a few ways to get hands-on nursing experience right now: volunteering in a hospital, taking a first aid course, or joining a Future Nurses club, if your school has one. These are all great options that will be discussed further on, but you have a wider range of options than this. You're almost certain to find one that's right for you . . .

IN YOUR SCHOOL

Future Nurses Club
You may be able to get your first experience of the nursing profession while gaining practical skills right in your own high school. Past students with an interest in nursing may have teamed up with a teacher or counselor to form a Future Nurses club. If so, you may find the club—similar to Future Farmers or Future Teachers clubs—very helpful in terms of hands-on learning *and* motivation. After all, it's easier to take on volunteer projects and push yourself to study harder when you have the support of others who share your goals. Together, you and the other future nurses will probably visit facilities such as hospitals and nursing schools, do some volunteer work to practice practical skills, and enjoy guest speakers with careers in the field of nursing.

But what if your school doesn't have a Future Nurses club? If you're really sold on the idea—and if you can sell it to a few other classmates—why not start your own club? That may sound daunting, but all you really need to start a Future Nurses club is some prospective members, a teacher or counselor to act as adviser, a place to hold regular meetings, and your principal's permission. With students and faculty working together, you can plan creative activities for the club and publicity to attract more members.

HOSA

If you are taking health occupations classes in high school, you are probably already familiar with HOSA or VICA. These are national organizations specifically for vocational students—and if your school is affiliated with either or both, they can be a real boost to your future in nursing.

Health Occupations Students of America (HOSA) has been working since 1976 "to promote career opportunities in the health care industry and to enhance the delivery of quality health care to all people." HOSA is an integral part of the health occupations curriculum in its member schools. One of its most visible activities is the annual Competitive Events Program, held at the state and national levels. Qualifying HOSA participants compete in many skill, leadership, and related events, including CPR/First Aid, Medical Spelling and Terminology, and Practical Nursing. HOSA also sponsors an annual National Conference. Remember, to participate in HOSA events, you must work with your school, so speak to a teacher or counselor about your interest in the organization. More information is available at http://www.hosa.org.

VICA

The Vocational Industrial Clubs of America (VICA) works with trade and technical students as well as those in health occupations, but like HOSA, it works through schools and in their curricula. Also like HOSA, VICA has a highly visible annual competition, called the Skills USA Championships. It's a large event with local, state, and national levels of competition in such categories as Basic Health Care Skills, Health Occupations Knowledge, and Practical Nursing. Work with your school officials to determine if VICA is an option for you. Their Web site can be found at http://www.vica.org.

Blood Drive

Whether or not your school already has formal clubs for prospective nurses, there is one experience of practical nursing that is possible at almost every school: a blood drive. Usually managed by the Red Cross, blood drives are often sponsored by Key Clubs, student councils, and even individual students with great organizational abilities. By getting involved in the sponsorship of a blood drive, you'll get to work with medical professionals, witness the functions they carry out, and perform a real service for people in need of blood transfusions.

Volunteering

Hospitals. Outside of school programs, the most familiar way to gain practical nursing experience is probably volunteering at a hospital, also called "candy-striping." This is so popular because it's available in most communities and so intimately connected to the work of professional nurses. Naturally, the specifics of volunteering vary among hospitals, but there is a lot of common ground. First of all, you can expect to undergo some kind of training—a couple of hours or a couple of days—to work on the skills needed in your particular duties. You will probably have to wear some kind of uniform and a name badge to make your identity and position clear to both patients and staff. And you will have to commit yourself to a schedule, so that the hospital can depend on you. Beyond this, the actual days and hours you work and the specific duties you perform are between you and the hospital's volunteer coordinator.

Your options will depend upon the size of the hospital you choose and whether it is a general, children's, or veterans' hospital. One rather exceptional example of a hospital for Denver-area residents to consider is The Children's Hospital of Denver, which has nearly 1,900 people in its Association of Volunteers. The Junior Volunteers program is for those ages thirteen to eighteen, who work in departments throughout the hospital and in fund-raising campaigns. Those working directly with patients may help feed them, make their beds, take their temperatures, or assist their nurses by running errands, fetching supplies, and doing some paperwork. These are some of the most basic duties in nursing, and if you enjoy performing them, it's a good indication that you're on the right career path. If you are in the Denver area, you may contact The Children's Hospital of Denver via the Association of Volunteers at 303-861-6887 or via the Web site at http://www.tchden.org.

Incidentally, volunteering at a children's hospital or in the children's ward of a general hospital could be your stepping stone to a career as a pediatrics nurse. It's obviously a great way to get experience in that specialty and it will also rid you of any illusions you might have about caring for sick children. Some people considering pediatrics nursing think it's mainly about seeing cute kids and healing a few bumps and bruises. But even as a volunteer, you will find that children are demanding patients and that many of their illnesses and injuries are as serious and distressing as those that afflict adults.

Hospices. Hospices and similar institutions generally care for the terminally ill and those with specific diseases such as cancer or AIDS. They sometimes accept teen volunteers, too, so if you are familiar with one in your area, get in touch to see if you can be of service. You would gain basic nursing skills and also see if that is the kind of work environment you might like to work in professionally. One special example of this kind of volunteer opportunity is the Human Service Alliance.

HUMAN SERVICE ALLIANCE

The Human Service Alliance (HSA) is a nationally recognized organization that offers volunteer opportunities for high school students who want to serve the community while gaining experience in caring for the ill and incapacitated. The HSA is a nonprofit, volunteer-run organization; it has no paid staff. There are four main areas on which the HSA focuses: care and comfort of the terminally ill; respite care of the developmentally disabled; mediation of conflicts; and health and wellness of the chronically ill or recovering injured. No previous experience is necessary; all volunteers receive suitable training before they begin. High school students who live nearby can volunteer for a few hours each week, helping out with such activities as bookkeeping and fundraising as well as patient care. Students from around the country can arrange to volunteer full-time for a minimum of two weeks up to an entire summer. Full-time volunteers usually work with the terminally ill "guests" at the HSA's Center for the Care of the Terminally Ill. Such students volunteer fifty to sixty hours per week helping to care for guests around the clock; their duties may also include such vital tasks as preparing specialized diets and cleaning the center to provide a pleasant and sanitary environment. Those volunteers who honor their time commitments are usually provided with room and board at the HSA, but they must pay for their own transportation and incidental expenses.

Contact the HSA about volunteering at least two months in advance of the date on which you would like to start. The HSA has no formal requirements for its volunteers, but clearly this is demanding work which must be undertaken by those who are mature, loving, generous, and willing to work as part of a team. For more information about the HSA, its mission, and its volunteer opportunities, contact the Human Service Alliance.

Human Service Alliance
3983 Old Greensboro Road
Winston-Salem, NC 27101
Tel: 910-761-8745 or 800-455-6463
Fax: 910-722-7882
Email: inquiry@hsa.org

Nursing Homes. If previous experiences in your life have taught you that you get along with the elderly especially well, consider volunteering at a nursing home or other facility for the aged. In terms of nursing duties, you can usually be of as much use in these institutions as in hospitals or hospices. You can also offer your own companionship to the elderly, who may rarely get to socialize with younger people or who may be far away from their own children and grandchildren. You can also work with older people by participating in such programs as Visiting Pets and Meals on Wheels. These may be community-run services or you might access them through a local church. If these experiences confirm that you have a particular talent for working with the elderly, you might consider specializing as a geriatrics nurse.

CPR and First Aid
Finally, you should seriously consider taking a class in CPR or First Aid—or both. Your local Red Cross, YMCA, or hospital most likely offers this kind of training for a reasonable fee. CPR and First Aid skills are obviously of great importance to every nurse, in every specialty, in every employment situation, and you can get a head start. But before you actually become a nurse—and even if you eventually decide not to go into nursing at all—CPR and First Aid courses will allow you to react promptly and effectively to medical emergencies around you. How should you react if a teacher faints in class? What should you do if a classmate cuts herself badly in industrial arts? If you've taken the proper courses, you'll know.

Besides CPR and First Aid, the Red Cross offers a number of courses and programs that are worth exploring. They can provide you with the training needed to educate your peers and your community about HIV/AIDS, staying healthy, swimming and water safety, and how to respond to disasters. Each local Red Cross office has different programs available, so call the one nearest you to see what it has to offer teens. You might also want to check out the Red Cross' extensive Web site—which will help you locate the office in your area—at http://www.redcross.org.

PREPARING FOR NURSING: PERSONAL QUALITIES

You've probably come to the conclusion that most of the activities listed in this section have required the important personal qualities of a nurse we discussed earlier: dedication, responsibility, maturity. If so, you're absolutely right! All of the volunteer activities involve other people depending on you, and you'll need all of these qualities to measure up to your duties. Volunteering probably won't be easy at first, but persevering and learning how to make the situation better can help you become more mature, dedicated, and responsible.

The camps and study programs listed here can do the same. Taking college-level courses, working on science projects with people you've just met, living away from home—possibly in another state—these are very different from volunteer work, but they demand the same qualities of you. And they can bring those qualities out of you.

A final personal quality that has been evident throughout this section—and is evident throughout the field of nursing—is, of course, generosity. The giving of yourself to ensure the well-being of others is a quality you can practice anywhere and everywhere. If you would like to make an especially generous effort in connection with nursing, you might consider doing charity work. It need not take much time: helping out with the March of Dimes once a year will help combat birth defects. Distributing red ribbons to raise AIDS awareness may take a few hours on a single Saturday. But doing such things genuinely helps others and puts your own good intentions to work right now. The March of Dimes, various AIDS prevention groups, and many more charitable organizations are as close as your phone book.

If one or more of the suggestions in this chapter sound interesting to you, put pen to paper or pick up the phone and start dialing. These suggestions are just the tools that *you* must put to use. It's your career, your future—and only you can plan it and start working toward it. Contact some of the organizations listed here or similar ones in your area and speak to the person who coordinates the program that interests you. Often, they will take some time to speak with you about your career goals, your personal situation, and how you might fit into their program. If that program doesn't seem right for you, ask for suggestions about other opportunities and organizations. Take the initiative and find the best way to explore your future in nursing right now.

Surf the Web

FIRST

You *must* use the Internet to do research, to find out, to explore. Short of an "all nursing, all the time" channel on TV, the Internet is the closest you'll get to what's happening now all over the place. This chapter gets you started with an annotated list of Web sites related to nursing. Try a few. Follow the links. Maybe even venture as far as asking questions in a chat room. The more you read about and interact with nursing and nurses, the better prepared you'll be when you're old enough to participate as a professional.

One caveat: you probably already know that URLs change all the time. If a Web address listed below is out of date, try searching on the site's name or other key words. Chances are, if it's still out there, you'll find it. If it's not, maybe you'll find something better!

ADDISON-WESLEY NURSING NETWORK

http://heg-school.awl.com/awnrsng

Provided by the publishing firm of Addison-Wesley Longman, this site offers features useful to prospective nurses, nursing students, and professional nurses alike. As you would expect from a publisher, there is a catalog of all the nursing books they offer and an on-line order form. But even if you're not interested in buying, it's worth reading over the sample chapters of their newest books.

Other features of the site include a calendar of nursing events and workshops and links to job listings, nursing organizations, and the latest health care news. There are tips on surviving nursing school and even a "Virtual Nursing Classroom" where you can test your knowledge with Vital Signs Jeopardy. The Addison-Wesley Nursing Network is definitely worth a look.

AMERICAN ASSOCIATION OF COLLEGES OF NURSES (AACN)

http://www.aacn.nche.edu/index.html

The AACN describes itself as the national voice for nursing education programs, and on a first glimpse this site may seem too academic. But delve into the right sections, and you'll see that it contains some precious nuggets for students considering a future in nursing. In fact, one of this site's most useful tools is specifically aimed at nurses-to-be. Under a section called Prospective Nursing Students, you'll find a lengthy, informative article that debunks some misconceptions about the field and explores the changing job market. There's also a financial aid fact sheet and a directory of AACN's more than five hundred member schools.

> This extremely well-organized site also includes a schedule of upcoming conferences and seminars. If academics is your thing, go ahead and read AACN's newsletter and other related publications online. The emphasis is on government affairs and college accreditation, topics more of interest to the professional nurse.

AMERICAN RED CROSS

http://www.redcross.org

The Red Cross is mentioned several times in the "Get Involved" section for its blood drives, CPR and First Aid courses, and the training it provides to young people who want to educate others about various health and safety issues. On its Web site, at the ARC Link, you'll find all of these options and many more explained in detail. There is a helpful little feature which allows you to type in your zip code and get contact information for the Red Cross office nearest you, so you can get involved right away.

> This site, which is both extensive and easy to use, also gives you an interesting history lesson via its Red Cross Museum, and puts you in touch with other humanitarian organizations that share its commitment to helping others. The American Red Cross has been an integral part of the country's health and safety efforts since 1881—it has a lot to offer you as you explore the field of nursing and it deserves a look.

ASSOCIATION OF OPERATING ROOM NURSES (AORN ONLINE)

http://www.aorn.org:80/

Though the old-fashioned title of operating room nurse lingers, these professionals would prefer to be called perioperative registered nurses to more accurately reflect their duties before, during, and after surgery. You'll learn about their responsibilities and also find clear descriptions of various nursing roles such as scrub nurse, circulating nurse, RN first assistant, and patient educator at this well-designed, frequently updated site.

But this site isn't for nurses only. The AORN sees itself as an advocate for patients, and they've developed "Surgery Center: A Patient's Place" (http://www.aorn.org/PATIENT/intro.htm), an incredibly user-friendly resource of patient-centered information relating to surgery and the surgical process. If someone among your family or friends is preparing for a surgery, point them here for excellent information they might not easily find elsewhere.

As the professional organization for perioperative nurses, the AORN has more than 350 chapters in all 50 states and throughout the world. Student nurses can join for a reduced rate to be eligible for scholarships and grants and to receive the usual member perks.

CHILDREN'S HOSPITAL OF DENVER ASSOCIATION OF VOLUNTEERS
http://www.tchden.org/aov/

While you can find plenty of hospitals with volunteer programs on the Web, the Children's Hospital of Denver, profiled in "Get Involved," stands out for its user-friendly home page and for the longevity and success of the program itself.

This site provides some background on the association, which boasts almost 1,900 volunteers who log over 160,000 hours of service a year. The volunteers work in various capacities: holding and comforting infants, offering support to parents, bringing specially trained dogs to provide animal-assisted therapy, and raising funds for a respite garden.

For many of the younger volunteers (the youngest is thirteen), this volunteer work is a way to "test-drive" a future career in medicine or nursing. If you've been doing volunteer work for a local hospital—or would like to—this site might strike a chord.

COOL NURSING SITE OF THE WEEK (CNS)
http://www.odyssee.net/~fnord/nurselink.html

It's mighty hard to predict just what you'll find here. As the name suggests, this site will point you to a "cool" nursing site each week. And just what constitutes cool? The Webmaster (a full-time nursing student) writes that he tries to seek out "hidden sites" related to nursing that will surprise visitors. For instance, the site recently showcased the Band-Aids & Blackboards health education project, which aims to sensitize schoolchildren to what it's like to grow up with medical problems.

You can also visit the archives where every CNS winner from the beginning of time is listed in reverse chronological order. This site stands out for doing more than just posting a list of links. Each linked site has a pithy, one- or two-sentence description so you can decide for yourself if it's "cool" enough to warrant a visit.

If you enjoy this site and don't want to miss a single week, sign up to receive an email when new sites are chosen. (CNS promises that updates are sent once a week only and that you will not be added to any other mailing lists.)

CRITICAL CARE NURSE SNAPSHOTS
http://www.nursing.ab.umd.edu/students/~jkohl/scenario/opening.htm

Does the idea of becoming a critical care nurse in a hospital setting appeal to you? This site is made up of interactive case scenarios involving nurses who must make informed decisions at the bedside. Each case study makes *you* a part of the critical thinking process involved in assessment, diagnosis, management, and follow-up of a problem. It's easy to navigate, and the descriptions of patients' medical conditions are clearly written and understandable even to the layperson. There are even photographs to give you a look at a critical care unit and its hypothetical patients.

The first scenario puts you in the shoes of an experienced nurse working the night shift with three new nurses, when you find that Patient A is experiencing difficulty breathing and Patient B has chest pain. What would you do first? Make the right decision and you'll be commended; make a poor choice and you'll be sent back to rethink the situation.

Obviously, some of the medical details go beyond your current knowledge base, but this is an excellent way to test your instincts about nursing.

HEALTHWEB: NURSING
http://www.lib.umich.edu/hw/nursing.html

An impressive, collaborative effort of the Taubman Medical Library, the School of Nursing at the University of Michigan, and the HealthWeb project, this site is a heavyweight of nursing information.

Under the mantle of Career Information, you can link to the *Occupational Outlook Handbook* in its entirety, or (if you're a rational person) just click on the nursing sections already plucked out for you, such as working conditions, employment, training, job outlook, earnings, and related occupations. You might be encouraged to read here that employment of registered nurses is expected to grow rapidly through the year 2005, with many of the new jobs in home health, long-term, and ambulatory care.

In the Communication section, you'll find information and email addresses for a number of on-line nursing discussion groups. If there's a particular field of nursing that piques your interest, the specialized discussion groups are a good place to gain insight into the field. The Education section has links to international and U.S. nursing schools on the Internet. Other pages will link you to nursing school newsletters and other nursing journals. If you're the kind of person who believes there's no such thing as too much information, you'll love this site.

INSIGHT ONLINE: HUMAN ANATOMY
http://www.innerbody.com/htm/body.html

Whether you need a little help in your anatomy class or just want to do some exploring on your own, this site offers an interesting way to explore the systems of the human body. You have your choice of ten systems: cardiovascular, digestive, endocrine, female reproductive, lymphatic, male reproductive, muscle, nervous, skeletal, and urinary.

Every image in every system features points on which you can click to see the name of selected body part. Click again for a definition or description of that part. Some animation showing the parts in action is also available. This site is simple and straightforward enough for users with little background in human anatomy.

THE INTERACTIVE FROG DISSECTION
http://curry.edschool.Virginia.EDU/go/frog/

Dissect a frog on-line? If you've got the amphibian, a scalpel, and an Internet connection, you're ready. With color photographs and downloadable QuickTime movies, this Web site just might conjure up the aroma of formaldehyde.

The site was designed to provide a step-by-step interactive tutorial for use in high school biology classrooms. It can also be used as a preparation tool or as a substitute for an actual laboratory dissection. The complete dissection is divided into Introduction, Preparation, Skin Incisions, Muscle Incisions, and Internal Organs. In each section, procedures for dissection are clearly described and presented in photographs.

The creators of this site invite your feedback to make it even better. Anybody interested in anatomy will want to check it out, as will students who are thinking of authoring their own tutorial Web site.

JOURNAL OF NURSING JOCULARITY (JNJ)
http://jocularity.com/

It takes a certain kind of person to be tickled by jokes about bodily functions. According to this site, it takes a nurse.

The Web edition of this quarterly journal for nurses is filled with satire, true stories, and cartoons written, illustrated, edited, and published entirely by nurses. And with over one hundred well-organized, easy-to-navigate on-line pages, you probably won't run out of laughs.

Since much of the humor in *JNJ* derives from making fun of stressful nursing situations, you'll get a pretty accurate idea of what things stress nurses out. Recent feature articles included "The Nurse's Bladder" and "How to Irritate a Nurse." You'll also find a section devoted to true stories of student nurses in the trenches. And here's a new tongue twister that you'll see a lot of in *JNJ*—psychoneuroimmunology. Basically, what the word means is that laughing is good for your health.

Some of this humor definitely has a "you needed to be there" flavor, but it does reveal a refreshingly silly side of health care.

KAPLAN'S GUIDE TO NURSING AND THE NCLEX
http://www.kaplan.com/nclex/

A commercial enterprise sponsored by Kaplan Educational Centers, this site provides some interesting information for students entering the nursing field. The section on careers provides a promising glimpse at future opportunities. For instance, did you realize that entry-level salaries for nurses with an undergraduate degree are the highest in the nation when compared to every other four-year degree?

A great deal of this site is written for students who have already earned a bachelor's degree in nursing and are preparing to take the NCLEX exam, the standardized test that evaluates for competency to practice nursing. In the careers section, for example, you'll find information about using a nursing degree as a stepping-stone to advanced career paths such as nurse administrator, nurse attorney, or nurse clinician. Though you're probably still mulling over how to get through nursing school, it never hurts to plan ahead.

Learn and Serve America

http://www.cns.gov/learn/index.html

Learn and Serve America is a grants program that funds "service-learning" programs; that is, community activities that complement classroom studies. The aim of these programs is to help students increase their academic skills while improving the quality of life in their communities. As part of a college-level program in New York, for instance, nursing students helped run a health center serving low-income people. The students gained practical experience while also meeting the health needs of those who couldn't otherwise afford health care. In one high school, students planned, prepared, and served lunch in a homeless shelter on a weekly basis as part of their health education class.

While much of this site is directed at school administrators rather than students, it does showcase several of the projects students are working on nationwide. You can search the on-line state-by-state directory to see if schools near you are involved. If your school doesn't currently participate in a program like this, you might consider forwarding this site's URL to your high school principal.

Men in Nursing

http://www.geocities.com/Athens/Forum/6011/

Don't make the mistake of thinking nursing is just for women. According to this site, the world's first nursing school was in India in 250 BC, and at that time, only men were considered "pure" enough to become nurses.

History buffs and equal opportunity enthusiasts will find some fascinating tidbits here, ranging from details about the Byzantine empire to an account of Juan de Mena, the first nurse in what was to become the United States. On a down note, this site-in-progress is utterly lacking in visual appeal. At this point it's entirely text-based and laborious to read through, page by page.

If you're intrigued by the history of nursing, this site certainly merits a visit. Even those of you who are more interested in the here and now will find modern-day factual data here, as well as contact information for the American Assembly for Men in Nursing (AAMN).

My Future

http://www.myfuture.com/

You want to become a nurse, but perhaps a four-year college just isn't in the cards for you. This colorful site aims to help new high school graduates "jump-start their lives" with information about alternatives to four-year colleges, such as military opportunities, apprenticeships, and technical or vocational colleges. In the hefty military career database, you'll find dozens of job descriptions for positions like medical care technician, physician assistant, registered nurse, and pharmacist.

While the site is divided into three main sections—My Career, My Money, and My World—most of the useful stuff is in the career section. For instance, you'll find the Industrial Strength Career Toolkit, with tools for doing self-exploration about career choices. You can take a career interest quiz to find out if you have a realistic, investigative, artistic, social, enterprising, or conventional work personality.

You'll also find some good info in the money section. For instance, play the Money Game for a chance to see what your spending decisions will cost you (without dropping any real greenbacks). Or visit the section called Searching for Dollars to get a handle on the financial aid process.

NATIONAL GERONTOLOGICAL NURSING ASSOCIATION (NGNA)

http://www.nursingcenter.com/people/nrsorgs/ngna/

This site is sponsored by the first and only specialty organization dedicated to gerontological nursing. If you are interested in improving the nursing care of the elderly, this is a specialty you've probably already considered.

So the good news is that this organization exists. The bad news is that its current Web site is little more than a well-written bulletin about NGNA's offerings. The on-line information is limited to descriptions of *Geriatric Nursing,* a professional journal; *New Horizons,* a bimonthly newsletter; NGNA's local chapters; and other membership benefits. You'll have to make a phone call to receive more in-depth information.

But wait: there's a glimmer of hope. The site now has an interactive message area where members can exchange news and information. Perhaps there's more in store for this site in the future.

NATIONAL SERVICE SCHOLARS

http://www.cns.gov/scholarships/index.html

Have you been an active volunteer in your community—perhaps at the local hospital, homeless shelter, or nursing home—for over a year? If so, your volunteer work could add up to $1,000 toward your nursing education.

This Web site will clue you in on the National Service Scholars program, which is a way for schools and communities to recognize young people for outstanding volunteer service and help them to continue their education. High school juniors and seniors who have performed community service for at least a year can be nominated for a $500 National Service scholarship, matched with $500 by a local organization.

Here's the catch: your high school principal is responsible for submitting the application. Assuming you're on good terms with your principal, you could download all the information from this site, drop it in his or her mailbox, and then start dropping hints.

NURSEWEEK
http://www-nurseweek.webnexus.com/

Nurseweek, an on-line magazine, operates like a professional clipping service for nurses. Right on the home page, you'll read today's medical news updates. Recent headlines, for example, featured the pros and cons of proposed tobacco regulations, nurses pushing for minimum staffing levels, and the court-upheld ban on physician assistants performing abortions.

This is a comprehensive, appealing, and eclectic read for those in the nursing or health care field. One of *Nurseweek's* regular features is an on-line survey (recently about physician-assisted suicide), where you can simply answer "yes" or "no" or submit a full letter to the editor. In subsequent editions of the magazines, readers can see the survey results on-line. *Nurseweek* also publishes lengthier articles about the nursing profession, and recently, a special career guide for student nurses. In that same issue you could read some practical tips for coping with stress and an interview with the author of a book about life support.

And what Web site would be complete without links to other Web sites? That's right, you'll find many links to other nursing resources—such as education and job sites—here.

NURSINGNET
http://www.nursingnet.org/

Could you use some advice about nursing careers or nursing school from someone who's already been there? NursingNet is the place to look. Its centerpiece is a new on-line mentoring program connecting nurses and nursing students from around the world to discuss their jobs and studies with one another. Just fill out an on-line application to become a participant.

For less formal mentoring, there are several chatrooms and discussion groups available within the site. The Virtual Nurse chatrooms, however, are disappointing, consisting of little more than people asking, "Is anyone else in this room?" A section called NursingNet forum is more substantive, with nurses and students seeking and providing advice on specific topics.

If you're shopping for colleges, there's a section with handy links to nursing schools around the world. Or maybe you want to know more about individual nursing specialties: click on sections dedicated to maternal and newborn nursing, geriatric nursing, emergency nursing, and more. You will also find a quick link to WholeNurse, an affiliated site that takes a more holistic view of nursing, with articles on alternative medicine and prayer used in the hospital.

THE NURSING STUDENT WWW PAGE
http://www2.csn.net/~tbracket/htm.htm

Here's a site designed for and by nursing students from around the country. Read the editors' bios on-line and you'll get a sense of just how diverse the nursing field is. But read on and you might also get the impression that these editor/student nurses are busy with things other than maintaining Web pages. Some of the sections could really benefit from more frequent updating. The list of links to Web sites of interest to nursing students, for instance, is on the skimpy side.

Still, there's a lot to recommend this site. The section called Study Help, for instance, is a fun read. It's the on-line equivalent of an upperclassman taking you under wing and giving straightforward advice on test-taking, "attitude adjustment," getting the most out of your books, using technology, and thriving in clinicals.

Want to know if your sense of humor is compatible with your future classmates and co-workers? Then check out the section called Nursing Humor for a laugh (or not). Putting all fun aside, the Math Skills section posts new problems monthly to help student nurses who want to sharpen their drug calculation skills.

NURSINGWORLD
http://www.nursingworld.org/

The American Nurses Association's site, NursingWorld, promises "nursing's future at your fingertips." That's a tall order, and this behemoth site doesn't always live up to it. While there's a ton of information to be found here, much of it is devoted to member information for three affiliate organizations—the American Academy of Nursing, the American Nurses Credentialing Center, and the American Nurses Foundation.

One of the most lively sections of NursingWorld is the *Online Journal of Issues in Nursing,* published in partnership with Kent State University's School of Nursing. Recent articles included "Clueless in the Land of Managed Care" and "Viva La Difference," an essay in support of keeping two types of advanced practice nurses—clinical nurse specialists and nurse practitioners.

Visit NursingWorld's news kiosk for timely health care news. NursingWorld also has a smattering of information about ethnic minority fellowships, international nursing, and legislative news. And once you're in nursing school, you'll find the searchable reading and reference rooms extremely useful.

THE PRINCETON REVIEW
http://www.review.com/

This site is everything you want in a high school guidance counselor—it's friendly, well informed, and available to you night and day. Originally a standardized test preparation company, the Princeton Review is now on-line, giving you frank advice on colleges, careers, and of course, SATs.

Students who've spent their summers and after-school hours volunteering at a clinic or hospital will find good tips here on how to present those extracurricular activities on college application forms. There's a handy link to *Time*'s interactive guide, "The Best College for You," which discusses costs, admissions, and alternatives to four years of college. If you're looking for contact with other students who are weighing their options, too, link to one of the discussion groups on college admissions and careers.

Two of the Princeton Review's coolest tools are the Find-O-Rama, which creates a list of schools based on the criteria you type in, and the Counselor-O-Matic, which reviews your grades, test scores, and extracurricular record to calculate your chances of admission at many colleges.

RN STUDENTS HOME PAGE
http://members.aol.com/RNstudents/index.html

An abundance of sites like this one seem to have sprung up. An enterprising nursing student somewhere decides there should be a resource page to help other students find the valuable stuff on the Web. This site doesn't provide much in the way of editorial content, but it does get you right to links that are organized in an easy-to-grasp fashion.

Current links include the World Health Organization, Medscape (which allows you to search research papers), nursing organizations, nursing schools on the Internet, nursing career information, Centers for Disease Control, the on-line nursing magazine *ADN/RN Concepts,* and more.

STUDENT NURSE INFORMATION CENTER
http://glass.toledolink.com/~ornrsg/

You'll discover in nursing school that the cost of buying textbooks each semester or quarter can add up quickly. This site features a Book Exchange marketplace for student nurses who want to sell, buy, or trade books online with other students across the country. You'll need specific information to post or search for a book here, including the name of the book, author, edition, and ISBN number.

Other than the Book Exchange, this site is largely a sluggish aggregate of links to other sites. These links include nursing specialties, nursing journals and organizations, formulas and conversions, hospitals on-line, schools and educational resources, nursing newsgroups, and a chat feature.

U.S. NURSING CAREER TITLES
http://www.amideast.org/pubs/aq/aqnrsttl.htm

Don't expect to be overwhelmed by colorful, interactive multimedia here. But if your head is swimming with the initials LPN, RN, and NP, you might find this site an informative respite from the more all-inclusive sites. This Web page, which is actually just a reprint of a magazine article, does exactly what its name suggests—concisely defines the various titles used in the nursing industry.

For instance, do you know what it takes to become a nursing assistant, psychiatric aide, or registered nurse? Which position requires more education and training, public health nurse or nurse practitioner? Under each job title, there's information about the length of on-the-job training needed, licensing and education requirements, and a brief description of job responsibilities. If you're just familiarizing yourself with the job prospects in nursing and health care, take three or four minutes to visit this site.

| | |
Read a Book

FIRST

When it comes to finding out about nursing, don't overlook books. (You're reading one now, after all.) What follows is a short, annotated list of books and periodicals related to nursing. The books range from fiction to personal accounts of what it's like to be a nurse, to professional volumes on specific topics, such as death and dying and dealing with doctors. Don't be afraid to check out the professional nursing journals, either. The technical stuff may be way above your head right now, but if you take the time to become familiar with one or two, you're bound to pick up some of what is important to nurses, not to mention begin to feel like a part of their world, which is what you're interested in, right?

We've tried to include recent materials as well as old favorites. Always check for the most recent editions, and, if you find an author you like, ask your librarian to help you find more. Keep reading good books!

BOOKS

Alfaro-Lefevre, Rosalinda, and Marcia E. Blicharz. *Drug Handbook: A Nursing Process Approach.* Reading: Addison-Wesley Publishing Co., 1992. A useful reference for nurses, nursing students, and anyone interested in the types of medications nurses handle and administer.

Anderson, Peggy. *Nurse.* New York: Berkley Books, 1979. A major best-selling account of the life of Mary Benjamin, RN. A remarkable and entertaining book about the life of a nurse—her thoughts and feelings, daily duties, and life-and-death experiences. Required reading for all first-year nursing students.

A Nurse You Should Know

It seems like nurses in the 1990s have more career options than ever before. Registered nurses can serve in hospitals, nursing homes, clinics, doctors' offices, or the armed forces. They can specialize in pediatrics or geriatrics, or work as surgical nurses. As far back as the 1940s, however, one nurse named Cherry Ames worked in all of these positions—and more!

The catch is that Cherry is the fictional heroine of a series of young adult novels, begun in 1943 and written by Helen Wells and Julie Tatham. In 27 books, Cherry pursues a career from Student Nurse to Veterans' Nurse to Mountaineer Nurse and beyond. Though often compared to fictional sleuth Nancy Drew because of her ability to solve mysteries, Cherry Ames is first and foremost a nurse. Each book illustrates the many different challenges and rewards of the nursing profession, through Cherry's own experiences and those of the patients, doctors, and other nurses she meets.

The Cherry Ames Nurse Stories naturally encourage readers to consider the dozens of career paths within nursing. But more than this, the series impresses upon every reader what it means to be a nurse, and what it takes to be a good one. As important as formal training and qualifications are to Cherry, she is constantly aware that the single most important requirement for nursing is the desire to serve others. Whether in imminent danger as Army Nurse or exhausted after long and arduous shifts as Chief Nurse, Cherry Ames knows that her first responsibility is always the health and welfare of her patients, not her own comfort and contentment. While the circumstances surrounding nursing careers have changed dramatically since Cherry's time, her qualities and ideals are as important as ever.

The Cherry Ames Nurse Stories are no longer in print, so you won't find them in bookstores. But if you're looking for enjoyable books, some insight into nursing, and even a little inspiration as you consider entering this demanding profession, look for Cherry Ames in your school or public library. All twenty-seven books in the series were published in the United States by Grosset and Dunlap. There is an additional book by Helen Wells, *Cherry Ames' Book of First Aid and Home Nursing* (1959), now a bit dated, of course, but endorsed in its time by the National League for Nursing.

Barnum, Barbara Stevens. *Spirituality in Nursing: From Traditional to New Age.* New York: Springer Publishing Co., 1996. Gives a thorough and readable overview of spirituality, cast as a component of nursing theory and practice. Addresses such major nursing issues as healing, religion, ethics, disease, and death.

Belkin, Lisa. *First, Do No Harm.* New York: Fawcett Books, 1994. An absorbing novel by a former New York Times correspondent about the inner workings of Hermann Hospital in Houston, Texas. Examines many profound and complicated questions about life and death.

Camenson, Blythe. *Nursing.* VGM Career Portraits. Lincolnwood: NTC Publishing Group, 1995. Offers excellent vocational guidance to the young reader, and covers a broad range of nursing issues and concepts.

Case, Bette, ed. *Career Planning for Nurses.* Albany: Delmar Publishers Inc., 1997. Useful, proactive tool for nurses at all levels. Discusses what

1. *Cherry Ames, Student Nurse.* Wells, 1943.
2. *Cherry Ames, Senior Nurse.* Wells, 1944.
3. *Cherry Ames, Army Nurse.* Wells, 1944.
4. *Cherry Ames, Chief Nurse.* Wells, 1944.
5. *Cherry Ames, Flight Nurse.* Wells, 1945.
6. *Cherry Ames, Veterans' Nurse.* Wells, 1946.
7. *Cherry Ames, Private Duty Nurse.* Wells, 1946.
8. *Cherry Ames, Visiting Nurse.* Wells, 1947.
9. *Cherry Ames, Cruise Nurse.* Wells, 1948.
10. *Cherry Ames at Spencer.* Tatham, 1949.
11. *Cherry Ames, Night Supervisor.* Tatham, 1950.
12. *Cherry Ames, Mountaineer Nurse.* Tatham, 1951.
13. *Cherry Ames, Clinic Nurse.* Tatham, 1952.
14. *Cherry Ames, Dude Ranch Nurse.* Tatham, 1953.
15. *Cherry Ames, Rest Home Nurse.* Tatham, 1954.
16. *Cherry Ames, Country Doctor's Nurse.* Tatham, 1955.
17. *Cherry Ames, Boarding School Nurse.* Wells, 1955.
18. *Cherry Ames, Department Store Nurse.* Wells, 1956.
19. *Cherry Ames, Camp Nurse.* Wells, 1957.
20. *Cherry Ames at Hilton Hospital.* Wells, 1959.
21. *Cherry Ames, Island Nurse.* Wells, 1960.
22. *Cherry Ames, Rural Nurse.* Wells, 1961.
23. *Cherry Ames, Staff Nurse.* Wells, 1962.
24. *Cherry Ames, Companion Nurse.* Wells, 1964.
25. *Cherry Ames, Jungle Nurse.* Wells, 1965.
26. *The Mystery in the Doctor's Office.* Wells, 1966.
27. *Ski Nurse Mystery.* Wells, 1968.

nurses can do to control their careers rather than succumb to the caprices of the marketplace.

Chambliss, Daniel F. *Beyond Caring: Hospitals, Nurses, and the Social Organization of Ethics, Morality, and Society.* Chicago: The University of Chicago Press, 1996. A challenging and engaging study of nurses' frustrations with their work and working conditions, and the role of ethics in nursing, drawing on research conducted in three hospitals between 1979 and 1990.

Cox, Helen C., Mittie D. Hinz, Mary Ann Lubno, and Susan Newfield, eds. *Clinical Applications of Nursing Diagnosis: Adult, Child, Women's, Psychiatric, Gerontic, and Home Health Considerations.* 3rd ed. A standard text for nursing patient-assessment, discussing a wide range of health patterns and complications and examining the role of the nurse in each case.

Craven, Ruth F., and Constance J. Hirnle. *Fundamentals of Nursing: Human Health and Function.* 2nd ed. Philadelphia: Lippincott-Raven Publishers, 1996. The consummate textbook for the first nursing course. Provides colorful, well-written, and thorough coverage of all basic nursing concepts, theory, and skills.

Croft, Jennifer. *Careers in Midwifery.* New York: Rosen Publishing Group, 1995. An overview of the history of midwifery, the categories of certification and training, birth settings, and career planning. Addresses midwives and the heath care debate.

Daly, Barbara J., ed. *The Acute Care Nurse Practitioner.* Springer Series on Advance Practice Nursing. New York: Springer Publishing Co., 1996. Upper-level but worthy collection of essays on the changing role of the nurse practitioner in the modern health care environment, addressing clinical skills, educational standards, and administrative functions.

Davis, Anne J., Mila A. Arosker, and Joan Liaschensko. *Ethical Dilemmas and Nursing Practice.* Paramus: Prentice Hall, 1997. A broad discussion of health care ethics and an outline of selected ethical approaches of nursing practice. A useful account of the moral dilemmas nurses typically face, from abortion to mental illness.

Decker, Phillip J., and Eleanor J. Sullivan. *Effective Leadership and Management in Nursing.* Reading: Addison-Wesley Publishing Co., 1996. Discusses nursing services, nurse administrators, nursing care, and nursing leadership. Useful and comprehensive.

Dossey, Barbara Montgomery, Lynn Keegan, and Cathie E. Guzzetta. *Holistic Nursing: A Handbook for Practice.* 2nd ed. Gaithersburg: Aspen Publishers, 1995. Describes the many ways in which nurses can complement traditional medical techniques with such alternative healing procedures as therapeutic touch, massage, guided imagery, and music.

Douglas, Ellen, and Elizabeth Spencer. *Apostles of Light: A Novel.* Banner Books. University: University Press of Mississippi, 1994. A novel about nursing home patients in the Southern United States, and the nurses who care for them.

Eliopoulos, Charlotte. *Gerontological Nursing.* 4th ed. Philadelphia: Lippincott-Raven Publishers, 1996. A readable and comprehensive basic gerontology text, focusing on health promotion and self-care. Clear, concise, and practically oriented, this text is the perfect guide to understanding and meeting the challenges of providing services to the elderly patients in a variety of settings.

Ellis, Rosemary. *Selected Writings of Rosemary Ellis: In Search of the Meaning of Nursing Science.* Edited by Joyce Fitzpatrick and Ida Martinson. New York: Springer Publishing Co., 1996. A wonderful collection of writings by one of nursing's most penetrating thinkers and treasured scholars.

Written with clarity, grace, and wit, this is an invaluable resource to nurse researchers, theorists, educators, and students.

Felice-Farese, Susan J., ed. *Poetic Expressions in Nursing . . . Sharing the Caring.* Long Branch: Vista Publishing, 1994. A unique collection of poetry relating to the nursing profession.

Frederickson, Keville. *Opportunities in Nursing Careers.* Lincolnwood: NTC Publishing Group, 1995. Offers good vocational guidance for a variety of nursing careers, exploring the financial benefits of each.

Friedman, Marilyn M. *Family Nursing: Research, Theory, and Practice.* Stamford: Appleton & Lange, 1997. A thorough survey of the educational requirements, procedures, and vicissitudes of family nursing.

Galanti, Geri-Ann. *Caring for Patients from Different Cultures: Case Studies from American Hospitals.* 2nd ed. Philadelphia: The University of Pennsylvania Press, 1997. Collection of case studies that illustrate how to avoid cross-cultural misunderstandings in the nursing workplace.

Henderson, Virginia. *A Virginia Henderson Reader: Excellence in Nursing.* Edited by Edward J. Halloran. New York: Springer Publishing Co., 1995. An inspiring collection of essays discussing anything from the importance of being a careful observer and the art and science of health assessment, to the role of research in nursing and the nurse's role in promoting health programs.

Keegan, Lynn. *The Nurse as Healer.* Lincolnwood: NTC Publishing Group, 1994. An accessible and thoughtful discussion of the psychological aspects of nursing. Discusses types of patient-nurse bonding, with an eye to teaching the nurse how to develop relationships with patients that are both personal and practical.

Kuhse, Helga. *Caring: Nurses, Women, and Ethics.* Boston: Blackwell Publishers, 1997. Discusses the often troubled relations between nurses and physicians, nursing ethics, and the nursing environment.

Leonard, Peggy C. *Building a Medical Vocabulary.* 4th ed. London: W. B. Saunders Co., 1997. Excellent guide to the language of health care. Teaches the fundamental word parts that are used as the "building blocks" of more complicated terminology.

Melosh, Barbara, ed. *American Nurses in Fiction: An Anthology of Short Stories.* History of American Nursing. New York: Garland Publishing, 1984. An excellent anthology that collects mostly recent fiction about the social life and customs of nursing in the United States.

National League for Nursing. *State-Approved Schools for Nursing L.P.N./L.V.N. 1995: Meeting Minimum Requirements Set by Law and Board Rules in the Various Jurisdictions.* Pub. No. 1. 37th ed. New York: National League for Nursing, 1995. Useful and very informative reference tool.

Perry, Anne Griffin, and Patricia A. Potter. *Clinical Nursing Skills and Techniques.* St. Louis: Mosby-Year Book, Inc., 1997. An introductory text outlining the fundamental skills and knowledge of nursing, from bathing patients to recognizing vital signs.

Peterson's Guides. *Peterson's Guide to Nursing Programs: Baccalaureate and Graduate Nursing Programs in the U.S. and Canada.* 3rd ed. Princeton: Peterson's, 1997. A fully updated, massive, and easy-to-use directory of the study and teaching of nursing. Absolutely indispensable.

Peterson, Veronica. *Just the Facts: A Pocket Guide to Nursing.* St. Louis: Mosby-Year Book, Inc., 1994. A quick and easy reference for beginning nursing students, filled with charts, graphs, outlines, and easy-to-read tables.

Rosenberg, Charles E. *The Care of Strangers: The Rise of America's Hospital System.* Baltimore: The Johns Hopkins University Press, 1995. An engaging and informative history of the hospital system, from the time of Thomas Jefferson to the present day.

Schneidman, Rose B., Susan S. Lambert, and Barbara R. Wander. *Being a Nursing Assistant.* Paramus: Prentice Hall, 1991. Fully approved by the American Hospital Association, this comprehensive, colorful book covers all the skills and procedures of the profession.

Selfridge-Thomas, Judy. *Emergency Nursing: An Essential Guide for Patient Care.* London: W. B. Saunders Co., 1996. A comprehensive, detailed, and honest overview of ER nursing.

Springhouse Publishing Co. *1,001 Nursing Tips & Timesavers.* 3rd ed. Springhouse: Springhouse Publishing Co., 1997. Excellent revised edition covers everything a nurse would need to know, from AIDS to computers to home health care. Includes appendices of most essential information for easy reference.

Springhouse Publishing Co. *Illustrated Handbook of Nursing Care.* Springhouse: Springhouse Publishing Co., 1997. Addresses every key nursing topic, and contains over five hundred illustrations along with charts and sample documentation forms. A total guide to the ins and outs of the nursing process.

Zawid, Carol Israeloff. *Sexual Health: A Nurse's Guide.* Real Nursing. Albany: Delmar Publishers Inc., 1994. A useful guide to sexual issues in the nursing workplace, from sexual hygiene and sexually transmitted diseases to sexuality and sexual behavior.

PERIODICALS

AJN, American Journal of Nursing. Published monthly by Lippincott-Raven Publishers, 227 East Washington Square, Philadelphia, PA 19106. An important and influential magazine, containing compelling articles and editorials, photo essays, and medical essays.

Computers in Nursing. Published bimonthly by Lippincott-Raven. Discusses the most up-to-date effects of computer technology on nursing theory and practice, particularly the changing learning environment of nursing science.

Home Healthcare Nurse. Published monthly by Lippincott Raven. Probably the most thorough journal of home health care nursing, providing strategies for assessing the health of homebound patients, and also for dealing with terminal illness, depression, and death.

Journal of Neuroscience Nursing. Published bimonthly by the American Association of Neuroscience Nurses, 224 North Des Plaines, Suite 601, Chicago, IL 60661. One of only two journals in the world specializing in neuroscience nursing; written and reviewed by practicing nurses.

Journal of Nursing Jocularity. Published quarterly by JNJ Publishing, Inc., at http://www.jocularity.com. Humorous publication for nurses and health care professionals, filled with satire, true stories, cartoons, and all-around funny stuff related to nursing and health care. Written, drawn, and edited completely by nurses and health care professionals.

JOGNN, Journal of Obstetric, Gynecologic and Neonatal Nursing. Published bimonthly by Lippincott-Raven. Features articles about the latest advances in childbearing, infant development, maternal psychology, labor technique, and much more.

Medsurg Nursing. Published monthly by Jannetti Publications, Inc., East Holly Avenue, Box 56, Pitman, NJ 08071-0056. The official journal of the Academy of Medical-Surgical Nurses, it provides readers with useful, multidisciplinary information about providing clinically excellent patient care in various surgical settings.

Nurse Educator. Published bimonthly by Lippincott-Raven. Discusses many issues of mentorship and professional role development in undergraduate and graduate nursing education. Offers a sense of what nursing educators look for in their students and peers.

Nursing History Review. Published annually by Springer Publishing Co., 175 5th Avenue, New York, NY 10010. Official journal of the American Association for the History of Nursing. Contains essays, editorials, articles, and reviews about nursing methods, theories, and movements.

Nursing Standard Online. Updated weekly by RCN Publishing Co., at http://www.nursing-standard.co.uk. Offers numerous interesting articles and abstracts from the most recent issue of *Nursing Standard*, a prominent British nursing journal.

Online Journal of Issues in Nursing. Published by the Kent State School of Nursing, PO Box 5190, Kent, OH 44240-0001, at   http://nursing-world.org/ojin.htm. An excellent forum for discussing and learning about pertinent issues in nursing, produced by one of the nation's finest nursing schools.

Ask for Money

By the time most students get around to thinking about applying for scholarships, they have already extolled their personal and academic virtues to such lengths in essays and interviews for college applications that even their own grandmothers wouldn't recognize them. The thought of filling out yet another application form fills students with dread. And why bother? Won't the same five or six kids who have been fighting over grade point averages since the fifth grade walk away with all the really *good* scholarships?

The truth is, most of the scholarships available to high school and college students are being offered because an organization wants to promote interest in a particular field, encourage more students to become qualified to enter it, and finally, to help those students afford an education. Certainly, having a good grade point average is a valuable asset, and many organizations that grant scholarships request that only applicants with a minimum grade point average apply. More often than not, however, grade point averages aren't even mentioned; the focus is on the area of interest and what a student has done to distinguish himself or herself in that area. In fact, frequently the *only* requirement is that the scholarship applicant must be studying in a particular area.

GUIDELINES

When applying for scholarships there are a few simple guidelines that can help ease the process considerably.

Plan Ahead

The absolute worst thing you can do is wait until the last minute. For one thing, obtaining recommendations or other supporting data in time to meet an application deadline is incredibly difficult. For another, no one does his or her best thinking or writing under the gun. So get off to a good start by reviewing scholarship applications as early as possible—months, even a year, in advance. If the current scholarship information isn't available, ask for a copy of last year's version. Once you have the scholarship information or application in hand, give it a thorough read. Try and determine how your experience or situation best fits into the scholarship, or even if it fits at all. Don't waste your time applying for a scholarship in literature if you couldn't finish *Great Expectations.*

If possible, research the award or scholarship, including past recipients and, where applicable, the person in whose name the scholarship is offered. Often, scholarships are established to memorialize an individual who was a religious studies major or who loved history, but in other cases, the scholarship is to memorialize the *work* of an individual. In those cases, try and get a feel for the spirit of the person's work. If you have any similar interests or experiences, don't hesitate to mention these.

Talk to others who received the scholarship, or to students currently studying in the same area or field of interest in which the scholarship is offered, and try to gain insight into possible applications or work related to that field. When you're working on the essay asking why you want this scholarship, you'll have real answers—"I would benefit from receiving this scholarship because studying engineering will help me to design inexpensive but attractive and structurally sound urban housing."

Take your time writing the essays. Make certain you are answering the question or questions on the application and not merely restating facts about yourself. Don't be afraid to get creative; try to imagine what you would think of if you had to sift through hundreds of applications—what would you want to know about the candidate? What would convince you that someone was deserving of the scholarship? Work through several drafts and have someone whose advice you respect—a parent, teacher, or guidance counselor—review the essay for grammar and content.

Finally, if you know in advance which scholarships you want to apply for, there might still be time to stack the deck in your favor by getting an internship, volunteering, or working part-time. Bottom line: the more you know about a scholarship and the sooner you learn it, the better.

Follow directions

Think of it this way—many of the organizations that offer scholarships devote 99.9 percent of their time to something other than the scholarship for which you are applying. Don't make a nuisance of yourself by pestering them for information. Follow the directions on an application, even when asking for additional materials. If the scholarship information specifies that you write for more information, write for it—don't call.

Pay close attention to whether you're applying for an award, a scholarship, a prize, or financial aid. Often these words are used interchangeably, but just as often they have different meanings. An award is usually given for something you have done: built a park or helped distribute meals to the elderly; or something you have created: a design, an essay, a short film, a screenplay, an invention. On the other hand, a scholarship is frequently a renewable sum of money that is given to a person to help defray the costs of college. Scholarships are given to candidates who meet the necessary criteria based on essays, eligibility, or grades, and sometimes all three.

Supply all the necessary documents, information, fees, etc. and make the deadlines. You won't win any scholarships by forgetting to include a recommendation from your history teacher or failing to postmark the application by the deadline. Bottom line: Get it right the first time, on time.

Apply early

Once you have the application in hand, don't dawdle. If you've requested it far enough in advance, there shouldn't be any reason for you not to turn it in well in advance of the deadline. You never know, if it comes down to two candidates, the deciding factor just might be who was more on the ball. Bottom line: Don't wait, don't hesitate.

Be yourself

Don't make promises you can't keep. There are plenty of hefty scholarships available, but if they all require you to study something that you don't enjoy, you'll be miserable in college. And the side effects from switching majors after you've accepted a scholarship could be even worse. Bottom line: Be yourself.

Don't limit yourself

There are many sources for scholarships, beginning with your guidance counselor and ending with the Internet. All of the search engines have education categories. Start there and search by keywords, such as "financial aid," "scholarship," "award." Don't be limited to the scholarships listed in these pages.

If you know of an organization related to or involved with the field of your choice, write a letter asking if they offer scholarships. If they don't offer scholarships, don't let that stop you. Write them another letter, or better yet, schedule a meeting with the president or someone in the public relations office and ask them if they would be willing to sponsor a scholarship for you. Of course, you'll need to prepare yourself well for such a meeting because you're selling a priceless commodity—yourself. Don't be shy, be confident. Tell them all about yourself, what you want to study and why, and let them know what you would be willing to do in exchange—volunteer at their favorite charity, write up reports on your progress in school, or work part-time on school breaks, full-time during the summer. Explain why you're a wise investment. Bottom line: the sky's the limit.

THE LIST

Air Force ROTC
Scholarships Branch
Maxwell AFB, AL 36112
Tel: 301-981-1110

Students with two years remaining at an accredited school of nursing may apply for financial support to complete their education; recipients must agree to serve for a specified period as an Air Force nurse. In addition, high school seniors intending to study nursing are eligible for four-year scholarships that also carry a service obligation.

Alpha Tau Delta
Scholarship Chair
PO Box 3566
Idyllwild, CA 92349
Tel: 909-980-3536

Members of an Alpha Tau Delta chapter are eligible for grants of up to $1,000 to help finance nursing training. Applicants must have strong academic records and demonstrate financial need. Deadline to apply is April 15.

Altrusa International Foundation
332 South Michigan Avenue, Suite 1123
Chicago, IL 60604
Tel: 312-427-4410

Women who hold a high school diploma or who are the sole support of a family are eligible for financial aid to help prepare for careers in health fields. Write for details.

American Association of Blood Banks
8101 Glenbrook Road
Bethesda, MD 20814
Tel: 301-907-6977

The Association awards scholarships to students who are enrolled in or accepted in a Specialist in Blood Banking Educational Program; scholarships of $1,500 are awarded to student winners of an annual essay contest. Apply by April 1.

American Association of Critical-Care Nurses
101 Columbia
Aliso Viejo, CA 92656
Tel: 714-362-2000

Educational Advancement Scholarships of $1,500 are open to current members or those enrolled full- or part-time in a nursing program. Applicants must be in their junior year and have at least one year of experience working in a critical-care unit. Apply by January 15.

American Association of Homes for the Aging
Education Scholarships
901 E Street, NW, Suite 500
Washington, DC 20004
Tel: 202-783-2242

Persons currently working as an aide in a nursing home who hope to earn the LPN or RN degree may apply for Nurse Education Scholarships of up to $1,000. Recipients must agree to work one year in a long-term health care facility for each year of aid received. Deadline to apply is July 15.

American Association of University Women Educational Foundation
PO Box 4030
Iowa City, IA 52243

Fellowships of $13,000 to $15,000 are available for women nurses to support research projects; write for details.

American Business Club
Box 5127
High Point, NC 27262
Tel: 910-859-2166

The Club offers three hundred awards annually of $500 to $700 to college juniors, seniors, and graduate students majoring in physical therapy, occupational therapy, or speech and hearing.

American College of Medical Practice Executives
104 Inverness Terrace
East Englewood, CO 80112
Tel: 303-799-1111

Richard Davis Scholarships of $1,000 are awarded to undergraduate or graduate students in ambulatory care or medical group management; deadline to apply is May 30. Write for details.

American Dietetic Association Foundation
216 West Jackson Boulevard, Suite 800
Chicago, IL 60606
Tel: 312-899-0400

Graduate scholarships ranging from $500 to $10,000 are available, as are undergraduate scholarships and internships of $500 to $1,000. Write for a complete list of awards.

American Holistic Nurses' Association
4101 Lake Boone Trail, Suite 201
Raleigh, NC 27607
Tel: 919-787-5181

The $500 Charlotte McGuire Scholarship is offered to nurses undertaking a holistic nursing program; applicants must be AHNA members for at least one year, and have a 3.0 GPA.

American Institute of the History of Pharmacy
Pharmacy Building
University of Wisconsin
Madison, WI 53706-1508
Tel: 608-262-5378

The Institute offers grants-in-aid to help graduate students who are students of pharmacy. Applicants may be enrolled at any college or university in the United States.

American Kinesiotherapy Association
PO Box 611, Wright Brothers Station
Dayton, OH 45409-0611
Tel: 800-326-0268

Kinesiotherapy majors at the undergraduate or graduate level may apply for scholarships of up to $500; candidates must be members sponsored by certified kinesiotherapists.

American Legion Auxiliary
1007 Murfreesboro Road, Suite 100
Nashville, TN 37217
Tel: 615-361-8822

Various state auxiliaries of the American Legion offer scholarships to help students prepare for nursing careers. Most require that candidates be residents of the state and associated with the organization in some way, whether as a child, spouse, etc., of a military veteran. Interested students should contact the appropriate local chapter for further information.

American Occupational Therapy Association, Inc.
PO Box 31220
Rockville, MD 20824-1220
Tel: 301-652-7590

Undergraduate and graduate students enrolled in occupational therapy programs are eligible for scholarships of $750 to $2,000. Applicants must be AOTA members.

American Physical Therapy Association
1111 North Fairfax Street
Alexandria, VA 22314
Tel: 703-684-2782

Physical therapy students in their final year of study are eligible for Mary McMillan Scholarships; awards are $1,000 for undergraduate and graduate students, and $5,000 for doctoral candidates.

American Respiratory Care Foundation
11080 Ables Lane
Dallas, TX 75229
Tel: 214-243-8892

Undergraduate scholarships of up to $1,250 are offered to second-year students in respiratory care programs; applications are accepted April 1 through May 30. In addition, $500 Morton B. Duggan, Jr. Memorial Scholarships are open to respiratory care majors, with priority given to applicants from Georgia and South Carolina.

American Society for Hospital Food Service Administrators
840 North Lake Shore Drive
Chicago, IL 60611
Tel: 312-280-6416

Dietary Products-Baxter Health Care Corporation Awards of $500 are open to ASHFSA members who are directors or assistant directors of food service in a health care institution. Applications are due February 1.

■ Archbold Memorial Hospital
Department of Education
Gordon Avenue and Mimosa Drive
Thomasville, GA 31799
Tel: 912-228-2830

Scholarships of up to $4,000 are available to students in their last two years of study in nursing, physical therapy, or another health field; recipients must agree to work for three years at the hospital following graduation.

■ Army ROTC Nursing Opportunities
PO Box 1688
Ellicott City, MD 21043
Tel: 800-USA-ROTC

Students going for a bachelor's degree in nursing may apply for scholarships paying tuition and some expenses; recipients must then serve with the Army for a specified number of years after graduation.

■ Association of Operating Room Nurses
Scholarship Board
2170 South Parker Road, Suite 300
Denver, CO 80231
Tel: 303-755-6300

Undergraduate, graduate, and doctoral students who are active or associate members of AORN are eligible for scholarships covering tuition and fees. Apply by May 1.

■ Baptist Hospital
1000 West Moreno Street
Pensacola, FL 32501
Tel: 904-434-4911

Nursing students who agree to later work for Baptist Hospital are eligible for scholarships of up to $1,500 to help finance training.

■ **Beta Sigma Kappa**
4500 Beechwood Road
College Park, MD 20740
Tel: 301-927-0508

Research grants of up to $600 are available for students working on a bachelor's degree in optometry. Applications due April 1.

■ **Business and Professional Women's Foundation**
2012 Massachusetts Avenue, NW
Washington, DC 20036
Tel: 202-293-1200

The New York Life Foundation awards $1,000 scholarships to women in health-related professions. Applicants must be at least thirty years old and within twenty-four months of completing an undergraduate degree program. Send a self-addressed, return envelope with two first-class stamps for details and materials. Applications are accepted October through April.

■ **Career Mobility Scholarships**
National Student Nurses Association Foundation
555 West 57th Street, Suite 1325
New York, NY 10019
Tel: 212-581-2211

Career Mobility Scholarships of up to $1,000 are open to LPN-LVNs enrolled in a program leading to licensure as an RN.

■ **Daughters of the American Revolution**
Scholarship Committee
1776 D Street, NW
Washington, DC 20006
Tel: 202-628-1776

Caroline Holt Nursing Scholarships are open to undergraduate students enrolled in a nursing program in the United States. Selection criteria include academic standing, financial need, and letters of recommendation; applicants need not be affiliated with DAR. Enclose a self-addressed, stamped envelope with your inquiry; deadline to apply is September 1.

■ **Diet Center, Inc.**
International Scholarship Program
220 South Second
West Rexburg, ID 83440
Tel: 208-356-9381

Ten $3,000 scholarships are awarded to junior or senior undergraduate students for study in nutrition or dietetics at an accredited institution. Applicants must have a 3.0 GPA; applications are due February 15.

■ District of Columbia League of Nursing
5100 Wisconsin Avenue, NW, Room 306
Washington, DC 20016
Tel: 202-244-0628

A $2,000 scholarship is offered to a registered nurse working toward a bachelor's or master's degree in nursing.

■ District of Columbia Public Schools
Division of Student Services
415 12th Street, NW
Washington, DC 20004
Tel: 202-724-4201

National Foundation March of Dimes Health Awards are open to students for study in health careers. Contact your school counselor for details.

■ Eckerd Drugs
PO Box 4689
Clearwater, FL 34618
Tel: 813-585-3995

The Pharmacy Assistance Program allows students who have completed two years of pre-pharmacy training to borrow $1,500. Applications are due May 1; write for further information.

■ Educational Advancement Scholarships for Generic Students
NSNA
555 West 57th Street
New York, NY 10019
Tel: 212-581-2211

To assist members of the American Association of Critical-Care Nurses (AACN) who are working on a degree in nursing. Registered nurses who are current members of the AACN or National Student Nurses' Association (NSNA) may apply if they have a cumulative grade point average of 3.0 or better and are enrolled in an accredited BSN program. This program is intended for students who are not yet licensed as an RN, although they may be licensed as an LVN or

LPN. Applicants must be entering their junior or senior year. At least 20 percent of these awards are allocated for ethnic minorities. The stipend is $1,500. The funds are sent directly to the recipient's college or university and may be used only for tuition or fees.

Epilepsy Foundation of America
4351 Garden City Drive
Landover, MD 20785
Tel: 301-459-3700

Bachelor's and master's students undertaking research projects related to epilepsy are eligible for $1,500 fellowships; medical students wishing to conduct similar research may apply for $2,000 awards. Apply by March 1.

Florida Hospital Association
PO Box B
Eustis, FL 32727

The Waterman Allied Health Scholarship of up to $2,500 is available for candidates seeking training in pharmacy, physical therapy, and other fields. Must work for six months in the Waterman Hospital for each $500 received.

Foundation for Nutritional Advancement
192 South Street, Suite 500
Boston, MA 02111
Tel: 617-728-9136

The Foundation awards scholarships to students majoring in nutrition or health sciences.

Foundation of the National Student Nurses Association
555 West 57th Street
New York, NY 10019
Tel: 212-581-2211

Several scholarships of $1,000 to $2,000 are open to NSNA members and non-members who are enrolled in an undergraduate nursing or pre-nursing program. Send a self-addressed, return envelope with two first-class stamps for details; apply by February 1.

Gwen Brieger Memorial Scholarship
American Association of Neuroscience Nurses
224 North Des Plaines, Suite 601
Chicago, IL 60661-1134
Tel: 312-993-0043 or 800-477-AANN

To provide funding to graduate and undergraduate students for the study of neuroscience nursing. This program is open to nurses who are seeking a degree or credential at the undergraduate or graduate level with a specialization in neuroscience nursing. The amount of the award depends on the availability of funds.

Health Resources and Services Administration
1010 Wayne Avenue, Suite 1200
Silver Spring, MD 20910
Tel: 301-495-0824

Scholarships of up to $800 are available for students in medicine, osteopathy, nursing, midwifery, and physician assistantship. Applications due March 20.

International Order of the King's Daughters and Sons
514 Colonial Avenue
Norfolk, VA 23507
Tel: 804-622-1583

Health Career Scholarships of up to $1,000 are awarded to students who have completed at least one year of study in physical or occupational therapy, pharmacy, or nursing. Send a self-addressed, stamped envelope for information; apply by April 1.

Kaiser Permanente of Northern California
Community and Government Relations
1950 Franklin Street, 3rd Floor
Oakland, CA 94612
Tel: 510-987-3289

Scholarship aid is available to support students enrolled in nursing programs and students pursuing nursing as a second career. Apply through the attending institution.

Kappa Epsilon Fraternity
2902 North Meridian
Indianapolis, IN 46208
Tel: 317-925-0778

Fraternity members in at least their sophomore year of pharmacy study are eligible for $500 Zada Cooper Scholarships; Wakeman Fellowships of $1,000 also are available for graduate study in pharmacy.

Kappa Kappa Gamma Fraternity
PO Box 2079
Columbus, OH 43216
Tel: 614-228-6515

Women in high academic standing who are college juniors, seniors, or graduate students are eligible for scholarships of $300 to $500 (undergraduate) or $300 to $1,000 (graduate) for study toward a degree in rehabilitation. Applicants need not be KKG members, but must attend a school with a chapter on campus. Send a self-addressed, stamped envelope for details.

Kentucky League for Nursing
PO Box 574
Murray, KY 42071

Nursing students are eligible for scholarships ranging from $200 to $1,000; applicants must have a high GPA and favorable references.

Marine Corps Scholarship Foundation
PO Box 3008
Princeton, NJ 08543
Tel: 609-921-3534

The Foundation helps children of marines and former marines with scholarships of up to $5,000 for study in nursing and other health fields. Applicant's total family gross income may not exceed $35,000.

Maternity Center Association
48 East 92nd Street
New York, NY 10128
Tel: 212-369-7300

The Association offers awards to persons who are already registered nurses who want to train to become nurse-midwives.

Methodist Hospitals Foundation
1211 Union Avenue
Memphis, TN 38104
Tel: 901-726-7880

The Dr. Leonard J. Vernon Scholarship of $1,000 is open to students accepted into a certified nurse anesthetist program. Recipients must seek employment at Methodist Hospitals of Memphis after completion of their training. Candidates need not be Methodist to apply.

Morrill Fund
Berea College CPO Box 2348
Berea, KY 40404
Tel: 606-986-9341

Interest-free scholarship loans are available to women intending to study nursing; priority is given to candidates from Southern Mountain states. Apply by May 10.

National Academy of Opticianry
10111 Martin Luther King, Jr. Highway, Suite 112
Bowie, MD 20720-4299
Tel: 301-577-4828

The Beverly Myers Achievement Award provides financial assistance to senior students currently enrolled in opticianry programs. The deadline for submitting dissertations is May 1. Students must be enrolled in an opticianry program accredited by the Commission of Opticianry Accreditation.

National Association of American Business Clubs
PO Box 5127
High Point, NC 27262
Tel: 910-888-6052

The Association awards $300 to $1,000 scholarships to students enrolled in physical, occupational, or music therapy, or speech and language pathology. Applications are due May 1; write for details.

National Association of Retail Druggists
250 Daingerfield Road
Alexandria, VA 22314
Tel: 703-683-8200

Student members of NARD enrolled in a pharmacy program may apply for loans of $1,000 to $2,000. Applicants must have completed the first two years of the program and have at least a 2.5 GPA. Membership cost is $15 per year; write for further information.

▓ National Association of School Nurses
PO Box 1300
Scarborough, ME 04074
Tel: 207-883-2117

The Lillian Wald Research Award is granted to NASN members to encourage research in the field of school nursing. Applicants must submit a research paper.

▓ National Athletic Trainers' Association
2952 Stemmons Freeway, Suite 200
Dallas, TX 75247
Tel: 214-637-6282

The Association offers $1,500 scholarships to graduate students pursuing careers as athletic trainers. Recipients must be NATA members; applications are due February 1.

▓ National Environmental Health Association
720 South Colorado Boulevard
South Tower, Suite 970
Denver, CO 80222
Tel: 303-756-9090

College juniors, seniors, and graduate students pursuing a degree in environmental health may apply for $400 to $1,000 scholarships; apply by February 1.

▓ National Foundation for Long Term Health Care
1201 L Street, NW
Washington, DC 20005-4014
Tel: 202-842-4444

The Foundation awards $500 to $1,000 scholarships to LPN and RN students interested in careers in long-term care; deadline to apply is July 31. For details, send a self-addressed, legal-size return envelope with two first-class stamps.

▓ National Foundation of Registered Nurse Education
1200 15th Street, NW
Washington, DC 20005
Tel: 202-659-3148

The Foundation awards $1,000 for training in an RN program for people working in a long-term care facility. Over fifteen awards are granted per year; apply by July 31.

National Foundation-March of Dimes
Office of Fellowships and Awards
1725 K Street, NW
Washington, DC 20006
Tel: 202-659-1800

Health Career Awards are provided to persons seriously intending to complete education in occupational therapy, physical therapy, medical social work, and other health professions. Candidates must be a citizen and legal resident of the United States, be a high school senior showing the greatest promise in special health fields who is graduating between January and July of the year entering college. Applicants must plan to enter a regionally accredited college or university in the fall as a full-time student, and intend to serve as a member of the health profession.

National Health Service Corps
Scholarship Coordinator
5600 Fishers Lane, Room 7-22
Rockville, MD 20857
Tel: 301-443-1650

National Health Service Corps Scholarships paying tuition and a monthly stipend of $767 are available for students of nursing, medicine, dentistry, or for certification as a physician's assistant. Recipients must practice one year in an underserved area for each year of aid received.

National Strength and Conditioning Association
PO Box 38909
Colorado Springs, CO 80937
Tel: 719-632-6722

The Challenge Scholarship is available to NSCA student members who have been members for at least one year. Application deadline is March 1. For requirements, call the NSCA.

Navy Recruiting

The Nurse Candidate Program provides financial support for students enrolled in a four-year nursing program; recipients must later serve on active duty with the Navy. This is one of several programs for nurses. Contact your local recruiter for complete details.

Non-Member Regular Scholarships
National Student Nurses Association Foundation
555 West 57th Street, Suite 1325

New York, NY 10019
Tel: 212-581-2211

Non-member Regular Scholarships of up to $2,000 are offered to students enrolled in a two- or four-year nursing or pre-nursing program; criteria include academic achievement, community involvement, and financial need.

Northwest Pharmacists Coalition Scholarships
PO Box 22975
Seattle, WA 98122
Tel: 206-746-9618

African-American students are eligible for financial aid to help them finance training in pharmacy. Applicants must be available for an in-person interview with the Coalition Scholarship Committee in the Seattle area at his or her own expense. Write for details.

NSNA Member Scholarships
National Student Nurses Association Foundation
555 West 57th Street, Suite 1325
New York, NY 10019
Tel: 212-581-2211

NSNA Member Scholarships of $1,000 to $2,500 are awarded to NSNA members enrolled in an undergraduate two- or four-year nursing or pre-nursing program; criteria include academic achievement, community involvement, and financial need.

Nurses Association Of the American College Of Obstetricians and Gynecologists
Department of Education and Research
409 12th Street, SW
Washington, DC 20024-2191
Tel: 800-673-8499

NAACOG members or associate members who have at least two years of experience in obstetrics, gynecology, and/or neonatology are eligible to apply for the $2,000 CIBA-GEIGY Fellowship. Candidates must be accepted into a program in nursing or midwifery.

Odwalla, Inc.
PO Box 0
Davenport, CA 95017
Tel: 408-425-4557

Women who are preparing for health careers are eligible for a scholarship offered by Odwalla. Write for details on the Femme Vitale Scholarship sending a self-addressed, stamped return envelope.

Oncology Nursing Foundation
501 Holiday Drive, Building 4
Pittsburgh, PA 15520
Tel: 412-921-7373

Registered nurses enrolled in an undergraduate or graduate program who are interested in oncology nursing may apply for $1,000 to $2,000 scholarships; apply by January 15.

Pharmaceutical Manufacturers Association Foundation
1100 15th Street, NW
Washington, DC 20005
Tel: 202-835-3400

Undergraduate research fellowships are available for pharmaceutical science students; graduate fellowships of $12,000 for doctoral candidates also are offered.

Pilot International Foundation
PO Box 5600
Macon, GA 31208
Tel: 912-743-7403

Undergraduate students preparing for careers working with people with disabilities are eligible for scholarships of up to $1,500 a year; apply through your local Pilot Club.

■ **Psychological Service Center**
   1212 Broadway, Suite 315
   New York, NY 10023

The Center provides four Mental Health Awards, one for $1,000 and one for $500 in each of two categories, senior and student. Candidates must submit a mental health paper or audio or visual project representing an original or innovative approach to an issue or problem relating to ethnicity and mental health.

■ **Quota International Fellowship Fund**
   1426 21st Street, NW
   Washington, DC 20036
   Tel: 202-331-9694

Fellowships of $500 to $3,000 are available for students preparing for careers working with the deaf or hearing impaired. Write for details.

■ **Rho Pi Phi**
   9280 Hamlin
   Des Plaines, IL 60016
   Tel: 708-635-9391

Members of student chapters of this pharmacy fraternity may apply for scholarships; selection is made within and by the individual chapters. Deadline is June 1; write for further information.

■ **Salzar Foundation**
   5 Averstone Drive East
   Washington Crossing, PA 18977

Grants of from $1,000 to $2,000 are offered to students in physical assistant training programs. Priority is given to students who have exhausted all other sources of assistance and still need financial aid.

■ **Suburban Hospital**
   Scholarship Committee
   8600 Old Georgetown Road
   Bethesda, MD 20814
   Tel: 301-896-3100

Scholarships of up to $5,200 a year are available to students in their last two years of study in nursing, radiology, and various technologies and therapies in exchange for a commitment to work at the hospital after graduation. Applications are due in April.

Texas Center for Rural Health
PO Drawer 1708
Austin, TX 78767
Tel: 512-479-8891

The Center links communities needing health personnel with students in health programs by providing financial assistance to students who agree to later work in that community.

Thompson Memorial Foundation
5373 Sky Valley Drive
Hixson, TN 37343
Tel: 615-877-3920

The Foundation awards undergraduate scholarships to students pursuing a degree in physical therapy, medicine, or religion. Applicants must have an interest in serving humanity and an above-average GPA; priority goes to candidates with a Christian background. Send a self-addressed, stamped envelope for information; apply by March 15.

Tyson Foundation
2210 Oaklawn
Springdale, AR 72762
Tel: 501-290-4000

Students who live in the area of a Tyson Foods operating facility are eligible for $200 to $1,000 scholarships to help finance college study in nursing. Apply by June 20.

U.S. Department Of Education
Rehabilitation Services Administration
400 Maryland Avenue, SW
Washington, DC 20202
Tel: 202-706-4766

The Rehabilitation Services Administration offers scholarship assistance to students who are preparing to become occupational or physical therapists. Write for details.

U.S. Public Health Service
Bureau of Health Professions
Division of Nursing
5600 Fishers Lane, Room 5C-14
Rockville, MD 20857
Tel: 301-443-4144

Nurse Anesthetist Faculty Fellowships are offered to faculty members pursuing advanced education in their field. Registered nurses preparing for teaching careers also are eligible for scholarships toward graduate study. Apply through the attending institution.

■ U.S. Public Health Service
National Health Service Corps
5600 Fishers Lane, Room 7-23
Rockville, MD 20857
Tel: 301-443-3744

The NHSC awards scholarships to students in nursing and physician assisting who agree to serve in a needy area after completing their education—one year for each year of aid received. Applications are available in December and due in late March.

■ U.S. Public Health Service
Recruitment Office
8201 Greensboro Drive, Suite 600
McLean, VA 22102
Tel: 800-221-9393

The Commissioned Corps of the PHS helps nursing students finance their final year of study in exchange for working for the Service after graduation. Write for details.

■ U.S. Public Health Service
Division of Associated and Dental Health Professions
5600 Fishers Lane, Room 8C-09
Rockville, MD 20857
Tel: 301-443-4144

Public Health Traineeships are open to students preparing for careers in health administration, health planning, environmental or occupational health, or another area in preventive medicine; apply through the attending institution.

■ U.S. Public Health Service
Indian Health Service Scholarship Program
12300 Twinbrook Metro Plaza, Suite 100
Rockville, MD 20852
Tel: 301-443-3744

The Health Professions Scholarship Program provides awards averaging $14,000 to students enrolled full-time in a nursing, pharmacy, optometry, social work, or health care administration program. Recipients must serve one year in an Indian health facility for each year of aid received.

U.S. Veterans Administration
Health Professions Scholarship Program
810 Vermont Avenue, NW
Washington, DC 20410
Tel: 202-535-7528

Students in their last two years of study in nursing, occupational or physical therapy are eligible for scholarships offering full tuition and a monthly stipend of $621. Recipients must later serve at least two years in a VA facility. Applications are due in May.

West Virginia Public Health Trust
PO Box 846
Charleston, WV 25323
Tel: 304-346-1438

Financial aid is available to professionals in medicine, nursing, public health, or research in drug addiction who agree to later practice in the state.

White Plains Hospital Center
Davis Avenue at East Post Road
White Plains, NY 10601
Tel: 914-681-0600

The Milstein Scholarship Program offers $5,000 to nursing students in their junior year.

Look to the Pros

The following professional organizations offer a variety of materials, from career brochures to lists of accredited schools to salary surveys. Many of them also publish journals and newsletters that you should become familiar with. Many also have annual conferences that you might be able to attend. (While you may not be able to attend a conference as a participant, it may be possible to "cover" one for your school or even your local paper, especially if your school has a related club.)

When contacting professional organizations, keep in mind that they all exist primarily to serve their members, be it through continuing education, professional licensure, political lobbying, or just "keeping up with the profession." While many are strongly interested in promoting their profession and passing information about it to the general public, these busy professional organizations are not there solely to provide you with information. Whether you call or write, be courteous, brief, and to the point. Know what you need and ask for it. If the organization has a Web site, check it out first: what you're looking for may be available there for downloading, or you may find a list of prices or instructions, such as sending a self-addressed, stamped envelope with your request. Finally, be aware that organizations, like people, move. To save time when writing, first confirm the address, preferably with a quick phone call to the organization itself, "Hello, I'm calling to confirm your address. . . ."

THE SOURCES

American Academy of Nurse Practitioners
LBJ Building
PO Box 12846, Capital Station
Austin, TX 78711
Tel: 512-442-4262
Web: http://npjobs.com/aanp

AANP offers a variety of free and inexpensive publications. Both *Scope of Practice* and *The Nurse Practitioner: A Primary Health Care Professional* describe the duties of a nurse practitioner and the education requirements. In addition to these on-line and print brochures, the Web site includes information on the national certification exam, as well as employment opportunities.

American Association of Homes and Services for the Aging
901 E Street, NW, Suite 500
Washington, DC 20004-2011
Tel: 202-783-2242
Web: http://www.aahsa.org

AAHSA offers a variety of free and inexpensive publications. *Considering a Career in Long-Term Care and Senior Housing*, 12 pages, available on-line, describes careers in the field of aging services and lists additional resources. The Web site includes contacts for state associations, grassroots networks, job information, publications, and FAQs.

American Association of Nurse Anesthetists
Bookstore
222 South Prospect Avenue
Park Ridge, IL 60068-4001
Tel: 847-692-7050, ext. 3009
Web: http://www.aana.com

AANA offers a variety of free and inexpensive publications, many available for ordering online. *Focus on Your Future*, 6 pages, describes the duties of certified registered nurse anesthetists, how to become a CRNA, educational and program requirements, and advantages of the profession. *Questions and Answers about a Career in Nurse Anesthesia*, 1 page, includes the most frequently asked questions and answers about the profession. *Council on Accreditation of Nurse Anesthesia Educational Programs: List of Recognized Educational Programs*, 10 pages, lists the programs by state, along with pertinent program information. *Certified Registered Nurse Anesthetists and the American Association of Nurse Anesthetists*, 8 pages, describes the impact of CRNAs on health care, their responsibilities, and their educational requirements. The Web site also includes information on the history of nurse anesthetist practice, education and accredited programs, and the qualifications and scope of practice of CRNAs.

American College of Nurse-Midwives
818 Connecticut Avenue, NW, Suite 900
Washington, DC 20006
Tel: 202-728-9860
Email: info@acnm.org
Web: http://www.midwife.org

ACNM publishes a variety of free and inexpensive publications: *A Career in Nurse-Midwifery: Your Ticket to the World,* 9 pages, includes a basic overview of the field, educational requirements, and sources of financial aid. *Education Programs Accredited by the ACNM Division of Accreditation,* 5 pages, lists schools offering certificate and master's nurse-midwifery programs. The Web site includes information on education and core competencies, financial aid, credentialing and licensure, history and philosophy of nurse-midwifery, and FAQs for students.

American Nurses Association
600 Maryland Avenue, SW, Suite 100 West
Washington, DC 20024-2571
Tel: 800-637-4ANA
Web: http://www.nursingworld.org

ANA offers *Career Letter,* 2 pages, which contains information on the nursing career. The Web site includes an online journal of issues in nursing, a publications catalog, and links to state nursing associations.

American Nursing Assistants' Association
PO Box 530374
Livonia, MI 48153-0374

Contact ANAA for career brochures and information on scholarships.

Association for Gerontology in Higher Education
1001 Connecticut Avenue, NW, Suite 410
Washington, DC 20036-5504
Tel: 202-429-9277
Web: http://www.aghe.org

AGHE offers a variety of free and inexpensive publications. Available free on-line is *Careers in Aging: Consider the Possibilities*, 12 pages, which discusses the field of gerontology, jobs and careers available, how to select a program, and how to find jobs in aging. Also available on-line is scholarship information, special resources for students, and a database of over one thousand gerontology programs.

Association of Operating Room Nurses, Inc.
2170 South Parker Road, Suite 300
Denver, CO 80231-5711
Tel: 303-755-6300
Email: dsmith@aorn.org
Web: http://www.aorn.org

AORN offers *Career Packet on Operating Room Nursing*, 55 pages, which discusses the profession, education and training, salaries, and other topics. The Web site includes information on scholarships and grants.

Commission on Graduates of Foreign Nursing Schools
3600 Market Street, Suite 400
Philadelphia, PA 19104-2651
Tel: 215-349-8767

CGFNS offers a variety of free and inexpensive publications. *An Overview of the Commission on Graduates of Foreign Nursing Schools*, 4 pages, provides an overview of the history and mission of the CGFNS. *CGFNS International Evaluator* is a quarterly report on nursing education and licensure.

Health Professions Career Opportunity Program
1600 Ninth Street, Room 441
Sacramento, CA 95814
Tel: 916-654-1730
Web: http://www.omhrc.gov/mhr2/progs/91c0970.htm

HPCOP offers a variety of free and inexpensive publications. *Health Pathways* is a quarterly newsletter containing timely information on health professional schools, admissions, postbaccalaureate and summer enrichment programs, financial aid, health careers, student health organizations, and health issues. *Financial Advice for Minority Students Seeking an Education in the Health Professions* discusses financial aid basics—costs, eligibility, availability, and resources. *The Many Roles of Nursing* includes information on career preparation, entry requirements, admission procedures, financial aid, and training.

■ **Midwives Alliance of North America**
PO Box 175
Newton, KS 67114
Tel: 316-283-4543
Web: http://www.social.com/health/nhic/data/hr0100/hr0170.html

Contact MANA for an information packet on a career as a midwife.

■ **National Association of Hispanic Nurses**
1501 16th Street, NW
Washington, DC 20036
Tel: 202-387-2477
Web: http://www.calumet.purdue.edu/public/finaid/nahn.htm

Contact NAHN for education and career information of particular interest to Hispanic nursing students, including scholarships, financial aid, and student services.

■ **National Association of Pediatric Nurse Associates and Practitioners**
1101 Kings Highway North, Suite 206
Cherry Hill, NJ 08034-1912
Tel: 609-667-1773
Email: info@napnap.org
Web: http://www.napnap.org

NAPNAP offers a variety of free and inexpensive publications. *Pediatric Nurse Practitioner School List*, 15 pages, lists for each institution programs and degrees offered, the academic schedule, and the minimum prerequisites. *Scope of Practice* ($2.50, available on-line) outlines basic functions and responsibilities of pediatric nurse associates and practitioners. The Web site includes FAQs, history of pediatric nurses and practitioners, and chapter links.

■ **National Black Nurses Association, Inc.**
1511 K Street, NW, Suite 415
Washington, DC 20005
Tel: 202-393-6870
Web: http://www.nbna.org

Contact NBNA for education and career information of particular interest to African-American nursing students.

■ **National Federation of Licensed Practical Nurses, Inc.**
1418 Aversboro Road
Garner, NC 27529
Tel: 919-779-0046
Web: http://www.nflpn.com

NFLPN offers *A Profile of Practical Nursing*, 6 pages, which describes what LPNs actually do, where they work, and what they earn. Also discusses the education required, school selection, licensure, continuing education, and general information about NFLPN.

National Health Council
1730 M Street, NW, Suite 500
Washington, DC 20036-4505
Tel: 202-785-3910
Web: http://www.nursingcenter.com/people/nrsorgs/ngna

NHC offers *200 Ways to Put Your Talent to Work in the Health Field* ($6.00), 35 pages, which lists job descriptions and education requirements for health professions ranging from art therapists and clinical chemists to nurse practitioners and physicians. It also lists sources of information on training schools and financial aid programs for health professions.

National League for Nursing
350 Hudson Street
New York, NY 10014
Tel: 212-462-0300

Contact NLN for career guidance materials and information on state approved schools of nursing.

National Student Nurses' Association, Inc.
555 West 57th Street, Suite 1327
New York, NY 10019
Tel: 212-581-2211
Email: nsna.net@internetmci.com
Web: http://www.nsna.org

NSNA offers *Is Nursing for You?*, 4 pages, which describes the various specialties, accreditation, how to choose a degree program, and personal requirements. The Web site includes information on the job market, scholarships, and resume writing and job hunting tips.

Oncology Nursing Society
Oncology Nursing Press
Department 1889
Pittsburgh, PA 15278-8847
Tel: 412-921-7373

ONS offers *Oncology Nurses Make a Difference: An Introduction to a Career in Oncology Nursing* ($1.25), which describes the various duties and responsibilities of an oncology nurse.

U.S. Department of Health and Human Services
Bureau of Health Professions, Division of Nursing
Room 9-35, 5600 Fishers Lane
Rockville, MD 20857
Tel: 301-443-6333
Web: http://www.hrsa.dhhs.gov/bhpr/bhpr.html

The USDHHS offers a variety of information. The Division of Student Assistance (301-443-4776) has information on health professions student loans (also available on-line). The grants management officer (301-443-6857) has information on professional anesthetist traineeships and professional nurse traineeships. There are also *Fact Sheets on the Division of Nursing Grant Programs*. Titles include *Advanced Nurse Education Grants, Nurse Practitioner/Nurse-Midwifery Program Grants, Nursing Education Opportunities for Individuals from Disadvantaged Backgrounds, Professional Nurse Traineeships, Nurse Anesthetist Traineeships, Nurse Anesthetist Education Programs*, and *Nurse Anesthetist Faculty Fellowships*.

Index